Spasticity Management
Rehabilitation Strategies

Linda A. Preston, OTR/L

Jeffrey S. Hecht, MD, F.A.A.P.M.R.

The American Occupational Therapy Association, Inc.

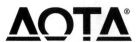

The American Occupational Therapy Association, Inc.
4720 Montgomery Lane
PO Box 31220
Bethesda, Maryland 20824-1220

Disclaimers
This publication is designed to provide accurate and authoritative information in regard to the subject matter covered. It is sold or distributed with the understanding that the publisher is not engaged in rendering legal, accounting, or other professional service. If legal advice or other expert assistance is required, the services of a competent professional person should be sought.

—From the Declaration of Principles jointly adopted by the American Bar Association and a Committee of Publishers and Associations

It is the objective of The American Occupational Therapy Association to be a forum for free expression and interchange of ideas. The opinions expressed by the authors are their own and not necessarily those of either the editors or The American Occupational Therapy Association.

ISBN 1-56900-117-0

Printed in the United States of America.

Table of Contents

Dedication

To our beloved spouses, Mark Durant Preston and Shelley August Hecht, without whose understanding, patience, love, and support, this project would have been truly impossible; our children, Ryan and Corey Preston and Robby, Sarah, and David Hecht, for providing us with joy and laughter; and our parents, Tom and Louise Anderson and Skip and Lynn Hecht, who taught us the value of continuing education and perseverance.

About the Authors

Linda Anderson Preston, OTR/L
Clinical Specialist
Patricia Neal Outpatient Therapy Center–Harriman
Roane Medical Center
Harriman, Tennessee
During the time that this book was written, Linda Anderson Preston was a Clinical Specialist at Synergistics, Inc., Oneida, Tennessee.

Jeffrey S. Hecht, MD, F.A.A.P.M.R.
Medical Director
Patricia Neal Rehabilitation Center at Fort Sanders Regional Medical Center/Covenant Health Care System
Associate Professor, Departments of Medicine and Surgery, University of Tennessee Graduate School of Medicine
University of Tennessee Medical Center
Knoxville, Tennessee

Preface

Spasticity can be a major limiting factor in a patient's ability to obtain normal movement and function. Unfortunately, spasticity management is often misunderstood in the health care community. Although there has been a marked increase in referrals of patients with spasticity problems from primary care physicians as a result of managed care, these physicians, as well as the occupational and physical therapists who subsequently care for the patients, are often not up to date on options for spasticity management. Therapists who are knowledgeable of current medical and surgical treatment options can be alert to situations warranting referral to specialists for consultation, and thus can be an integral component of a team effort to maximize treatment efficacy. Through this team effort, patients have a greater opportunity to attain their maximum level of function.

The need for information about spasticity management is greater now than ever before. Because monthly reports are often required to justify continued therapy and because inpatient length of stays are drastically shorter than they once were, occupational and physical therapists are a crucial link in ensuring that patient care is appropriately monitored. Although physician inpatient contact with patients who have experienced a cerebrovascular accident (CVA) has decreased in recent years, registered occupational therapists and certified occupational therapy assistants now treat these patients more frequently than patients with any other condition (American Occupational Therapy Association [AOTA], 1996a, 1996b). In addition, physical therapists also treat a high percentage of CVA patients. Patients with stroke are the second largest population treated by physical therapists (patients with low back pain are treated most frequently) (American Physical Therapy Association, 1998). Because nearly all patients with severe hemiplegia evolve to spasticity after passing through a flaccid stage, therapists must understand how to deal with this condition.

Occupational and physical therapists also have less direct contact with physicians than ever before, especially therapists who work in home health care, outpatient clinics, and extended care facilities. In

1996, a large percentage of registered occupational therapists (18.2%) and certified occupational therapy assistants (42.2%) listed skilled nursing homes or intermediate care facilities as their primary employment setting (AOTA, 1996a, 1996b). Primary care physicians can look to their therapist colleagues for the latest ideas in spasticity management. The therapist can play a triage role in initiating the referral process to other team members and monitoring treatment efficacy.

Until now, there has not been a comprehensive spasticity management book or journal article geared toward the needs of occupational and physical therapists. There are a plethora of innovations in nerve blocks, medications, and surgical options that therapists should be aware of. Also, the research reviewed in this book supports therapy treatment techniques that previously were based more on tradition than on rigorous study.

In addition, in the current managed care environment, health care dollars are sparse. Therapists and physicians must be able to work together to identify the most cost-effective treatment approaches.

This book will highlight theories used by occupational and physical therapists and present an organized description of treatment techniques, including physical agent modalities. Therapists should be able to use the book to refer appropriate candidates for nerve blocks, recognize adverse effects of oral and intrathecal antispasticity medication, be cognizant of common orthopedic procedures and refer possible candidates, and exhibit a general understanding of selective dorsal rhizotomy. Postnerve block and postoperative therapy protocols will be described and referenced.

Although this book is intended for occupational and physical therapists, the information presented should be useful for all health care professionals who care for patients with neurologic impairments. These health care professionals may include rehabilitation nurses, case managers, primary care physicians, pediatricians, and specialty physicians who are interested in the entire spectrum of spasticity management.

Acknowledgments

We are truly grateful to Robert Madigan, MD, for his review and valuable comments of the orthopedic surgery section of the manuscript, and to Patsy Grooms Cannon, PT, for her review and valuable comments in the casting section including the lower extremity cast figures. Special thanks go to Mary Ann E. Keenan, MD, Director of the Neuro-Orthopaedics Program at the Albert Einstein Medical Center and MossRehab in Philadelphia. Dr. Keenan provided, by personal communication, current information on upper extremity spasticity management. She also provided an advance copy of the chapter "Orthopaedic management of upper extremity dysfunction following stroke or brain injury" (Hisey & Keenan, 1999), which she wrote with Michael S. Hisey, J.D., for the 4th edition textbook, *Green's Operative Hand Surgery* (Green, Hotchkiss, & Pederson, 1999). We wish to thank Judy Hill, OTR, Audrey Yasukawa, MOT, OTR/L, and the Rehabilitation Institute of Chicago for sharing their upper extremity casting drawings. We are very grateful for personal communication input from Rehab Physicians of Knoxville, Tennessee; Helen Cohen, EdD, OTR; Fred Bennett, MD; Nancy King, PT; and Jenny Robison, PT. We thank Beth Asbeck for her original medical illustrations and manuscript reviews, Debra K. Allen for her artwork in redrawing the upper and lower extremities casting drawings, and Jennifer Griffith for assistance with syntax and format. We also wish to thank our patients who were willing to be photographed, and Myrna Cox, LPTA, for her photography. Garry Ogilvie, CO, Senior Practitioner at NovaCare, is appreciated for providing us with photographs of his progressive ankle–foot orthosis. Glenda Clark, Librarian of St. Mary's Medical Center, Knoxville, Tennessee, and the staff of Preston Medical Library at the University of Tennessee Medical Center–Knoxville are appreciated for their assistance. Robert Chironna, MD, J. Fred Znider, MD, and physicians of Knoxville Orthopedic Clinic are recognized for giving the authors liberal access to their libraries. Lorraine Pedretti, MS, OTR, is appreciated for offering publication advice.

This book was funded in part by Synergistics, Inc. of Oneida, Tennessee, and the Department of Surgery at the University of Tennessee Medical Center–Knoxville. We are grateful to Shriners Hospitals for Children, Lexington Unit, Lexington, Kentucky, for sharing rhizotomy evaluations and protocols and particularly appreciate the help of Tia Caldwell, OTR, and Chester Tylkowsky, MD. We acknowledge Patricia Neal Rehabilitation Center, Knoxville, Tennessee, for sharing its spasticity evaluation and casting procedures, and would like to thank the physical therapy staff of Patricia Neal Outpatient Center–Harriman and Roane Medical Center, Harriman, Tennessee, for their support. April Shepherd, Sheila Hicks, and Kathy Marshall are acknowledged for their word processing assistance. The senior author is grateful to her husband, Mark, for providing her with a peaceful week of writing in solitude at the Whitestone Inn, Kingston, Tennessee.

Chapter 1
Characteristics of Spasticity

The word spasticity is derived from the Greek word *spastikos*, meaning to tug or draw (Albright, 1992). Glenn and Whyte (1990) define spasticity as:

A motor disorder associated with a persistent increase in the involuntary reflex activity of a muscle in response to stretch. Four specific phenomena may be variably observed in the constellation of spasticity: hypertonia (frequently velocity dependent and demonstrating the "clasp-knife" phenomenon), hyperactive (phasic) deep tendon reflexes (DTRs), clonus, and spread of reflex responses beyond the muscle stimulated. (p. 2)

Patients with spasticity will often have difficulty initiating rapid movement and will have abnormally timed electromyographic activation of the agonist and antagonist (Katz, 1996). Although spastic muscles appear strong, they are actually weaker than normal muscles. Additionally, through the mechanism of reciprocal inhibition, a stronger spastic muscle will inhibit activity in its antagonist, thus accentuating the problem (Umphred, 1995).

Hyperactive tonic stretch reflexes (HTSR) have somewhat different characteristics than spasticity. HTSR are not velocity dependent, and no "clasp knife" is felt upon passive stretch. These reflexes are elicited through slow joint movement. The hypertonus persists as long as a passive stretch is maintained, secondary to the firing of group II muscle spindle afferents. HTSR occur in the flexor muscles in both upper and lower extremities and predispose the patient to flexion contractures. Both HTSR and spasticity are types of unilateral hypertonus (Little & Massagli, 1998). This book groups these two types of hypertonus together and refers to them as spasticity.

Neuroanatomy Review

It is important to differentiate between lower and upper motor neuron systems. The lower motor neuron system includes the following neural structures: cell bodies in the anterior horn of the spinal cord, spinal nerves, and the nuclei and axons of cranial nerves 3 through

1

10. Lower motor neuron dysfunction presents with flaccidity and decreased or absent deep tendon reflexes (DTRs) (McCormack & Pedretti, 1996).

Upper motor neuron syndrome (UMNS) affects any nerve cell body or nerve fiber in the spinal cord (other than the anterior horn cells) and all superior structures. This includes brain cells of both gray and white matter affecting motor function (excluding the cerebellum) and descending nerve tracts. UMNS presents with increased DTRs, due to lack of inhibition from superior centers.

Spasticity is merely one component of UMNS. Other signs of UMNS include presence of the Babinski sign, exaggerated cutaneous reflexes (including nociceptive and flexor withdrawal reflexes), and autonomic hyper-reflexia (the latter involving patients with spinal cord injury at level T-6 and above). An exaggerated nociceptive reflex can explain persistent pain not related to spasticity.

There are performance deficits noted in patients with UMNS. These include lack of dexterity, paresis, and fatigue (Young, 1994). Additionally, many UMNS patients have comorbidities such as sensory loss, ataxia, and perceptual and cognitive deficits that inhibit their function.

In order to understand the rationale of neurological treatment techniques, therapists must be familiar with the anatomy and physiology of the muscle spindle, including the mechanism of the DTR with and without gamma motor influence.

The muscle spindle is a complex encapsulated structure that lies deeply within the skeletal muscle structure. The muscle spindles lie parallel to the skeletal muscle (Figure 1). Each spindle houses four to six intrafusal fibers, and has sensory and motor innervation. The muscle spindle has two main functions: "monitor changes in length of a muscle, and the rate at which the length changes" (McCormack & Feuchter, 1996, p. 366 (Figure 2).

The DTR is easiest explained when describing the procedure of deformation of the patellar tendon with a reflex hammer: The reflex hammer strikes the patellar tendon, causing the quadriceps tendon to stretch. The primary stretch receptor is excited and sends impulses in proportion to the degree of deformation to the primary afferent (sensory) nerve. The primary afferent synapses with the alpha motor neuron. The alpha motor neuron sends a message to the motor end plate, resulting in skeletal muscle contraction (Werner, 1980).

The gamma motor neuron is the muscle spindle's motor innervation. It excites the spindle from upper motor neuron commands. If there is lack of inhibition from higher centers (resulting from UMN injury, infarct, or disease), the gamma motor neurons will receive too

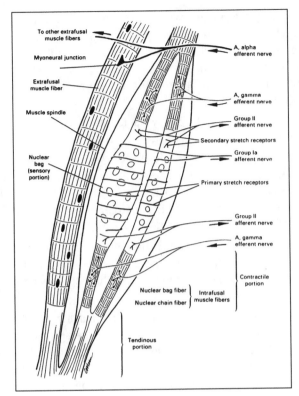

Figure 1. Muscle spindle depicting gamma motor neuron influence. From L. D. Lemkuhl and L. K. Smith (Eds.). (1983). Brunnstrom's *clinical kinesiology.* (4th ed.). Philadelphia: F. A. Davis. Reprinted with permission.

many contract messages (see Figure 2). The gamma motor neurons will make the contractile portion of the intrafusal fibers (polar region) contract. When these fibers contract, the central portion of the muscle spindle will stretch to the point where any additional input will set off a stretch reflex. Thus, hypertonicity (spasticity) results. Muscle

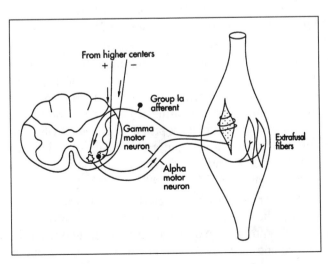

Figure 2. Muscle spindle depicting gamma motor neuron influence. From F. McCormack & F. Feuchter (1996). The Rood approach to treatment of neuromuscular dysfunction. In L. W. Pedretti (Ed.), *Occupational therapy practice skills for physical dysfunction* (4th ed., p. 366). St. Louis: Mosby-Year Book, Inc. Reprinted with permission.

spindle afferent nerves can facilitate spasticity in the spastic muscle, while inhibiting muscle tone in their antagonists. This is known as reciprocal inhibition. Impulses from the spastic muscle are sent to the spinal cord via the primary afferent nerve (McCormack & Feuchter, 1996). This nerve synapses with an inhibitory interneuron and inhibits tone in the opposing muscle.

The following definitions serve to clarify the functions of the individual parts of the muscle spindle:

1. *Intrafusal fibers*: There are two kinds of fibers, nuclear bag and nuclear chain. The polar ends of these fibers are contractile, however the central (equatorial) region of these fibers are noncontractile. The intrafusal fibers regulate tension in the muscle spindle.

2. *Gamma motor neuron*: This neuron is the motor innervation of the muscle spindle. It innervates the contractile ends of the muscle spindle. It receives inhibition or facilitation messages from upper motor neurons.

3. *Primary stretch receptor and its Group IA afferent nerve*: The receptor is located in the equatorial region of the spindle. It has a low threshold and can be excited by quick stretch, DTR testing, vibration, or any other action that causes elongation of the intrafusal fibers. It sends messages to the spinal cord via the Group IA afferent nerve.

4. *Secondary stretch receptor and its Group II afferent nerve*: It is also located in the equatorial region of the spindle, distal to the primary stretch receptor toward the tapered ends of the intrafusal fibers. The functions of the secondary receptor and the Group II afferent nerve have not yet been fully identified. They are believed to excite during a maintained stretch in maximal range (McCormack & Feuchter, 1996).

5. *Alpha motor neuron*: Innervates the extrafusal fibers of skeletal muscle, and resets after the muscle contracts. The cell body of the alpha motor neuron is in the anterior horn of the spinal cord. The alpha motor neuron receives information via the following structures or mechanisms: (a) Group IA and Group II afferent nerves, (b) "inhibitory postsynaptic potentials from interneuronal connections from antagonistic muscles and Golgi tendon organs, and (c) presynaptic inhibition initiated by descending fiber input" (Katz, 1996, p. 581).

In addition to understanding the muscle spindle, it is also important to comprehend the role of Golgi tendon organs (GTO). Golgi tendon organs are receptors located in the musculotendinous region in both the proximal and distal insertions. The GTO is felt to monitor tension in the tendon, and is believed to function as a protective mechanism via inhibiting contraction in the muscle in which it is located (Kisner & Colby, 1996). The GTO works with the muscle spindle to relay messages to higher centers. The higher centers then respond to this feedback by regulating tonicity and the action of the extrafusal muscles (Umphred, 1995). It is believed that the GTO can inhibit tone through the mechanism of autogenic inhibition. When excessive tension occurs in a muscle, the GTO fires and inhibits alpha motor neuron activity. This decreases tension in the skeletal muscle (Kinser & Colby, 1996). Refer to McCormack and Feuchter (1996) for further ways the GTO influences tone.

Peripheral nerves can be classified according to size: A, B, and C. A-size fibers are large myelinated fibers with a fast conduction rate. An example of an A-size fiber include gamma motor neurons. B-size fibers are medium sized, myelinated fibers that have a moderately fast conduction rate. An example of a B-size fiber is the branch of the alpha motor neuron. C-size fibers are either poorly myelinated or unmyelinated. They have the slowest conduction rate of all the nerve fibers. Examples of the C-size fibers include the exteroceptors; that is, pain, temperature, and touch (Umphred, 1995). Battery-operated brush and quick icing are felt to transmit impulses via the C-fibers (McCormack, 1996).

Types of Spasticity

There is a mild type of skeletal muscle spasticity caused by local factors, which can occur after trauma, is self-limited, and usually responds readily to treatment. It will not be reviewed. This book focuses on the two types of upper motor neuron spasticity: spinal and cerebral.

Spinal Spasticity

Spinal spasticity can result from spinal cord injury, spinal ischemia, degenerative myelopathy, transverse myelitis, spinal tumor, cervical spondylosis, multiple sclerosis, or familial spastic paraparesis or quadriparesis (Blumenkopf, 1997).

After spinal cord injury, the patient's tone is initially flaccid as a result of spinal shock. The affected extremities below the level of injury develop flexion and adduction tone (Young, 1994). With time, extensor tone develops and becomes the predominant type in the lower extremities (Katz, 1996). Spasticity is worse in incomplete spinal cord injuries (Blumenkopf, 1997).[1] Spinal cord hypertonicity

---

[1] It is interesting to note that the percentage of incomplete spinal cord injuries is increasing (National Spinal Cord Statistical Center, 1998).

can be extreme with severe episodes of muscle spasm (Pedretti, 1996).

An unusual pattern known as segmental myoclonus is sometimes seen in patients with spinal spasticity. It presents with ongoing repetitive spasms (Adams & Victor, 1989). Unlike other types of spasticity, it responds to anticonvulsant medicine (M. Weinstein, personal communication, February 19, 1998).

Cerebral Spasticity

Cerebral spasticity may stem from cerebral palsy, traumatic brain injury, stroke, anoxic event, brain tumor, metabolic disorder, or diseases of the brain. In multiple sclerosis, the spasticity stems from both spinal and cerebral disease (Blumenkopf, 1997).

In patients with cerebral spasticity, the degree of hypertonicity fluctuates as a result of changes in the patient's position. The antigravity muscles are affected; this generally includes the flexors of the upper extremities and extensors of the lower extremities (Pedretti, 1996; Young, 1994). Upper extremity flexion tone and lower extremity extension tone is the usual pattern seen in adult patients with stroke with hemiplegia. One should look for unusual problems when the pattern is different (such as lower motor neuron injuries or heterotopic ossification). Gravity has a major effect on spasticity, and thus on the methods of therapy used. For example, patients will usually have more tone when performing activities of daily living (ADL) in antigravity positions (the least amount of spasticity when recumbent; and the highest degree of tone upon ambulation). Serial casting will be easier when the patient is recumbent; however, if the patient sits up, the cast may become too tight due to the increase in spasticity.

Spastic diplegia in cerebral palsy presents itself with a lower extremity spasticity pattern similar to the adult person with hemiplegia, except in the hip and knee. Typically these children present with hip and knee flexion, as opposed to extension.

Considerations Before Spasticity Treatment

Before spasticity is treated, the therapist and physician need to closely evaluate the function of spasticity. Spasticity can have beneficial effects, such as maintaining muscle bulk, aiding in standing and transfers (Pedretti, 1996), and preventing deep vein thrombosis or osteoporosis. Treatment is necessary when spasticity interferes with ADL, gait, sleep, the patient's position in the wheelchair, or hygiene; or when it causes severe pain or contributes to the development of contractures or decubitus ulcers (Katz, 1996).

Spinal spasticity can increase as a result of painful or noxious stimuli. This stimuli often can be reduced with good medical care. (Eltornai & Montroy, 1990; Katz, 1988). Health care workers need to be aware of the more common factors that may worsen spinal spasticity: pressure sores, ingrown toenails, tight leg bags, confining shoes, tight clothing, blocked catheter, urinary tract infections, and fecal impaction (Eltorai & Montroy, 1990).

Review Questions

1. Describe the main differences between spinal and cerebral spasticity.

2. Excluding spasticity, what are the other performance deficits noted in upper motor neuron syndrome?

3. Draw a picture of the nuclear bag fiber of the muscle spindle, showing the gamma motor neuron, the Ia and II afferents, and location of their sensory endings. Explain how input is provided via the alpha motor neuron.

4. Quick icing and fast brushing affect what size peripheral nerve fibers: A, B, or C?

5. How can spasticity be helpful?

6. Name three indications or situations where spasticity should be treated.

Chapter 2
Occupational and Physical Therapy Spasticity Evaluation and Treatment

A thorough occupational and physical therapy spasticity evaluation would include the following subjective and objective measures: (a) the patient's and family's chief concerns about his or her spasticity, particularly how it affects function; (b) pain location and rating scale; (c) history of previous spasticity treatment with outcomes documented; (d) active and passive range of motion (ROM); (e) upper extremity coordination tests (f) muscle strength grades;[2] (g) usage of a spasticity quantification scale, such as the Modified Ashworth Scale (Bohannon & Smith, 1987); (h) spasm frequency score (if applicable); (i) effects of positioning and gravity; and (j) activities of daily living (ADL) assessment such as the Functional Independence Measure (FIM)™ instrument or the WeeFIM™[3] instrument rating system. Appendix A shows the adult spasticity evaluation form used at Patricia Neal Rehabilitation Center, Knoxville, Tennessee. Appendix B outlines the pediatric occupational therapy spasticity evaluation form used at Shriners Hospital in Lexington, Kentucky. Appendixes C, D, and E outline pediatric physical therapy spasticity evaluations. These are considered to be thorough pediatric spasticity evaluations that can also be used for nonsurgical pediatric patients.

Parts of the spasticity evaluation may need to be done serially to monitor and document progress. The use of a numbering system is helpful. Monthly progress summaries are usually required for patients

---

[2] Muscle strength is accurately evaluated when the patient is able to perform isolated movements. The therapist must keep a watchful eye for synergistic substitution patterns and associated reactions, as they can interfere with accurate strength assessment.

[3] FIM™ and WeeFIM™, instruments are trademarks of the Uniform Data System for Medical Rehabilitation, a division of UB Foundation Activities Inc., 232 Parker Hall, 3455 Main Street, Buffalo, NY 14214–3007.

in managed care as well as Medicare recipients. Objective documentation of progress can justify continued treatment, especially when spasticity interferes with function.

It is equally important to know when to stop treatment. When progress plateaus, the patient must be discharged from therapy.

An interdisciplinary team approach can be useful in most complex spasticity cases. The occupational and physical therapists play an important role among the following disciplines: neurology, neurosurgery, orthotics specialists, orthopedic surgery, and psychiatry. Many medical centers have developed spasticity management clinics in which various team members meet to formulate comprehensive plans of care.

Quantification of Spasticity

The five-step Ashworth Scale and the six-step Modified Ashworth Scale have been used to numerically rate spasticity in medical research more than any other scales in the past 10 years, based on the authors' English language MEDLINE search. The Ashworth Scale reads as follows (Ashworth, 1964):

1 No increase in tone

2 Slight increase in tone, giving a "catch" when affected part is moved in flexion or extension

3 More marked increase in tone: but limb easily flexed

4 Considerable increase in tone: passive movements difficult

5 Affected part rigid in flexion or extension

The Modified Ashworth Scale reads as follows (Bohannon & Smith, 1987):

0 No increase in muscle tone

1 Slight increase in muscle tone, manifested by a catch and release, or by minimal resistance at the end of the ROM when the affected part(s) is moved in flexion or extension

1+ Slight increase in muscle tone, manifested by a catch, followed by minimal resistance throughout the remainder (less than half) of ROM

2 More marked increase in muscle tone throughout most of the ROM, but the affected part (s) is easily moved

3 Considerable increase in muscle tone, passive movement is difficult

4 Affected part is in rigid flexion or extension

Some therapists and physicians find a three-step scale easier to use. Trombly and Scott (1977) outlined a three-step scale as follows:

1   Mild, if the stretch reflex occurs when the muscle is in a lengthened position

2   Moderate, if it occurs in the middle of the range

3   Severe, if it occurs when the muscle is in a shortened range

For a thorough review of other methods, scales, and factors regarding spasticity quantification, refer to Hinderer and Gupta (1996). Spasticity can fluctuate, even from hour-to-hour, day-to-day. There is some subjectivity with the currently available numerical rating scales.

Traditional Therapeutic Theoretical Approaches

The neurodevelopmental (NDT) approach developed by Bobath and Bobath is widely used by occupational and physical therapists and is accepted as effective (Bobath, 1978; Chakerian & Larson, 1993; Doraisamy, 1992; Glenn & Whyte, 1990). The NDT approach of evaluating tone involves observing and evaluating the patient's ability to adapt to specific movement patterns, as opposed to evaluating spasticity's effect on individual joint movement. In short, Bobath and Bobath advocated treatment techniques that attempt to normalize tone by inhibiting abnormal synergistic movement patterns while facilitating normal movement (Bobath, 1978).

Proprioceptive neuromuscular facilitation (PNF) was originated by Kabat at Kabat-Kaiser Institute in California. Kabat worked with physical therapist Margaret Knott to develop the PNF treatment approach. Dorothy Voss, physical therapist, joined their team at Kabat-Kaiser Institute in 1952. Knott and Voss wrote the first edition of their book, *Proprioceptive Neuromuscular Facilitation* in 1956. This book contains the PNF method of evaluating patient performance, noting the effects of spasticity on specific movement patterns. The PNF approach facilitates the development of normal movement patterns using rotational and diagonal movement components. Manual contacts, maximal resistance, and other facilitation techniques are incorporated in PNF (Knott & Voss, 1956).

Rood has completed research in techniques in sensory stimulation and how these techniques affect motor response (Rood, 1962). A few examples of Rood's techniques include icing, fast brushing, and heavy joint compression. Rood, as well as the Bobaths, Kabat, Knott, and Voss use developmental sequence as a foundation for their theories.

Brunnstrom, a physical therapist, evaluates adults with hemiplegia by focusing on the presence of limb synergies, primitive postural reflexes, and associated reactions. The Brunnstrom approach to treatment of hemiplegia recognizes that the patient progresses through six stages of recovery, promoting synergistic movement in the first three stages of recovery and working out of synergy in the last three stages (Brunnstrom, 1970).

Occupational and Physical Therapy Treatment

The most commonly practiced facilitation and inhibition techniques are listed below. The authors intend readers to use this as a quick reference for each technique, including neurological rationale, duration of effect, and contraindications. These techniques must be used in conjunction with a therapeutic activity and exercise program.

Facilitation Techniques

Fast brushing. Rood introduced use of a battery-operated brush over the skin or over a muscle to stimulate the C fibers, thereby stimulating the reticular activating system. Fast brushing can be done on the skin of the dermatome of the same segment that supplies the muscle needing facilitation (McCormack, 1996). The recommended duration is 3 to 5 sec for each area. After 30 sec, if there is no response, brushing should be attempted three to five more times. Effects of fast brushing peak at 30 to 40 min after stimulation (Trombly, 1983). One should monitor blood pressure when fast brushing on the face of patients with high cervical spinal cord or brain stem injury, as it can trigger autonomic dysreflexia (McCormack, 1996).

High frequency vibration. High frequency vibration is classified at a frequency between 70 to 300 cycles per second. Vibration stimulates the primary afferents in the muscle spindle, thereby causing a contraction of the muscle being stimulated, and inhibition of the antagonist (reciprocal inhibition) (Giebler, 1990; McCormack, 1996). The muscle or the tendon can be stimulated with vibration; the stronger effect would be on the latter. Vibration has been shown to be more effective than quick stretch. The length of the effect is typically 10 to 60 sec (Giebler, 1990). Vibration should not be performed longer than 2 min. Vibration can be used in conjunction with therapeutic activity. It can facilitate the patient's ability to sustain developmental postures, such as prone on elbows and all-fours weight bearing. There are contraindications to high-frequency vibration. It should be avoided near joints in children and not used at all in children under the age of 3 (McCormack, 1996). In adults, vibration has been shown to increase incoordination, rigidity, and tremors; her. use this technique with extreme caution (Giebler, 1990).

Tapping. Tapping over the desired muscle belly three to five times before or during active muscle contraction facilitates the primary afferents of the muscle spindle (McCormack, 1996).

Quick stretch. Quick stretch of a muscle activates the stretch reflex via stimulation of the primary afferents. The effect is immediate. The antagonist is inhibited (Trombly, 1983).

Resistance. Resistance stimulates both the primary and secondary receptors of the muscle spindle. Fast brushing and quick stretch can be administered before resistance (McCormack, 1996). Resistance is most commonly used to strengthen the antagonists to the spastic muscles. The senior author prefers cuff-weights over dumbbells in patients with flexion tone, as holding a dumbbell would facilitate finger flexion. Manual resistance is also effective.

Quick icing. Also known as C-icing, muscles can be facilitated using ice. Apply ice over the dermatomes of the same segment that supplies the muscle. Holding an ice cube in place for 3 to 5 sec is believed to begin to "stimulate posture, tonic responses via the C size fibers" (Trombly, 1983, p. 72). The effects of icing last 5 to 10 min. Therapists should avoid icing the trunk at L2 as this could lead to voiding, and S2–4 icing could lead to urinary retention (Trombly, 1983).

Skateboards. Forearm skateboards have shown widespread usefulness in strengthening 1+, 2– scapular, shoulder, and upper arm muscles. Therapists have used small toy cars as skateboards for radial or ulnar deviation and finger or thumb abduction or adduction facilitation (Figures 3 and 4), (E. Lawhorn, personal communication, June 1996).

Clinical Vignette

The first author treated a patient with traumatic brain injury who exhibited severe spasticity in his triceps and mild spasticity is his extensor digitorum communis 4 months postinjury. Upon initial evaluation, his passive elbow flexion was only 80°. The primary author strengthened his biceps with dumbbells, permitting him to only flex his elbow (therapist removed the weight from his hand, and passively extended his elbow). Over a period of 2 months, the biceps overpowered the spastic triceps, and he gained full elbow flexion. The triceps were strength-graded 4+ and the biceps were graded 5–. Bobath and Bobath caution against using heavy resistance with patients with neurological impairments, as this could promote associated reactions and feed into synergistic movements (Davis, 1996).

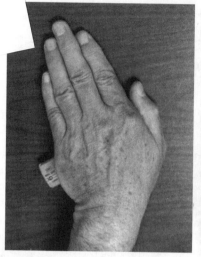 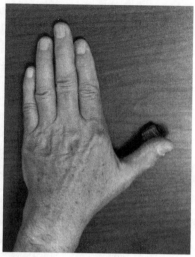

Figure 3. Toy car used as a skateboard to facilitate active ulnar deviation.

Figure 4. Toy car used as a skateboard to facilitate radial abduction of the thumb.

Inhibition Techniques

The techniques marked with an asterisk (*) are considered physical agent modalities.

***Sustained cold*.** Twenty minutes of application of a cold pack (skin cooled to 10°C has been shown to decrease the monosynaptic stretch reflex excitability (Giebler, 1990). It also has been shown to improve power in the antagonistic muscle groups (Katz, 1996).

Contraindications include "cryoglobulinemia, cold hypersensitivity or intolerance, rheumatic disorders including Raynaud's phenomenon, open wounds, circulatory deficits, and hypertensive patients" (Bonzani, 1997, p. 4).

Superficial heat. Heat has been found to have a short-term inhibitory effect on the muscle spindle. It can also provide pain relief and increase blood flow (Giebler, 1990). Stretching should immediately follow any type of superficial heat application. There are three types of superficial heat treatment:

1. Neutral warmth: Wrapping a body part or an extremity in a blanket has been shown to decrease muscle tone (McCormack, 1996).

2. Moist heat*: Wrap a hydrocollator pack in four to eight layers of terry cloth, and leave it on a spastic muscle for 20 min. Close supervision is recommended on patients with decreased sensation, aphasia, or confusion.

3. Paraffin bath*: The hand or foot is dipped in paraffin 7 to 12 times, covered with plastic, and then wrapped in a towel. This has been shown to be inhibitive (Giebler, 1990).

Contraindications to superficial heat include "insensate tissue, circulatory insufficiency, steroid dependency, or areas prone to bleeding" (Bonzani, 1997, p, 3).

Ultrasound.* When administered to a spastic muscle, ultrasound has been shown to increase blood flow and decrease tendon extensibility, thus relaxing the muscle. Typical treatment time is 5 to 10 min. The effects are short-lived, lasting 10 to 15 min (Giebler, 1990).

A specific target area for ultrasound application is the insertion of the subscapularis in the axilla (Figure 5). The subscapularis inserts into the lesser tubercle of the humerus. The subscapularis is the primary internal rotator of the shoulder. When this muscle is moderately or severely spastic it limits passive and active external rotation. The therapist can palpate the lateral aspect of the muscle in the axilla with simultaneous resisted internal rotation (N. King, personal communication, April 2, 1998). The authors recommend 6 to 12 treatment sessions of ultrasound followed by soft tissue mobilization and low load sustained subscapularis stretch before referral for a subscapularis phenol block.

Ultrasound is contraindicated in patients with "infections, malignancies, and metal implants" (Bonzani, 1997, p.6). Current thinking reveals metal implants may not be a problem with a moving technique or marked demineralization (Bonzani, 1997). Do not apply ultrasound over the heart or over demand pacemakers, over an

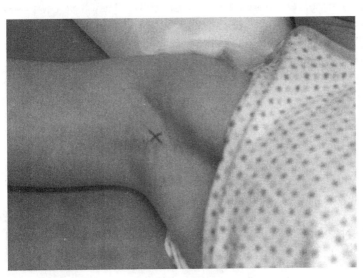

Figure 5. Ultrasound application to inhibit subscapularis insertion at the axilla.

unhealed fracture, on a "pregnant uterus, thrombophlebitis, insensate tissue, or epiphyseal areas" (Bonzani, 1997, p. 6). Avoid its use on children and over unhealed fractures. Avoid bony prominences when using continuous wave ultrasound (Bonzani, 1997).

Prolonged stretch. The primary author has had success gaining ROM by using joint mobilization techniques before prolonged stretch. Prolonged stretch helps prevent contractures and reduces tone for several hours. The reasons for a carry-over effect are "not completely clear but could be related to mechanical changes in the musculotendinous unit, as well as plastic changes that occur in the central nervous system" (Katz, 1988, p. 108). The duration of prolonged lower extremity stretch has been documented in a tilt table study. Standing on a tilt table for 15 min reduced lower extremity extensor spasticity in persons with spinal cord injury (Bohannon, 1993). The literature has not clearly specified time durations for upper extremity stretching. Static and dynamic splinting can also provide prolonged stretch. The authors have had success increasing passive ROM on an adult with head-injury with bilateral shoulder spasticity implementing 100-sec holds, five repetitions twice daily.

Air splints. Air splints have been shown to decrease spasticity by holding an extremity in inhibitive postures, maintaining pressure, and administering neutral warmth. The wearing schedule varies between 10 min to 2 hr (Giebler, 1990). The authors have had positive results in decreasing pain in spastic hemiplegic limbs after air splint application.

Elastic bandages. Bandages have a similar inhibitory effect of an air splint in providing and maintaining pressure and neutral warmth. These are made of cotton-rayon or cotton with elastic threads woven inside (Johnson & Vernon, 1992; Twist, 1985). They have been used with adolescents and adults with stroke and traumatic brain injury (Johnson & Vernon, 1992).

Transcutaneous electrical nerve stimulation* (TENS). High rate or conventional TENS have been used to inhibit spasticity. As with TENS used to relieve pain, the intensity is adjusted to produce a tingling sensation, without eliciting a motor response. This has been believed to inhibit tone via the "gate" theory by stimulating Group IA and Group IB fibers (Giebler, 1990).

Low rate TENS has also been shown to decrease tone. It is believed to stimulate slow conducting fibers such as Group IV (C-fibers). Please refer to Glenn and Whyte (1990, p. 131–133) for specific parameters.

TENS contraindications are the same as neuromuscular electrical stimulation (NMES) and are listed later in this chapter.

Other noteworthy inhibition techniques. Pressure on a tendinous insertion of the spastic muscle, gentle shaking or rocking, slow rolling, light joint compression, therapeutic bed positioning and rocking in developmental patterns have been shown to be inhibitive (McCormack, 1996).

Techniques That Can Either Facilitate or Inhibit

Weight bearing. Weight bearing has been shown to have both facilitating and inhibiting effects on the joint mechanoreceptors (Dee, 1969). A recent study at the Bobath Center in England determined that weight bearing had a positive effect on hand opening and development of prehension (Chakerian & Larson, 1993). Tilt table treatments decreased tone in lower extremities up to 4 hr in patients with spastic paraplegia (Giebler, 1990). There are numerous weight bearing positions. Common weight bearing postures used in neurorehabilitation include prone on elbows, "all fours," tall kneeling, standing, and sitting on a mat with weight bearing on the affected extremity.

Vestibular stimulation. Contingent on the rate of stimulation, vestibular stimulation can either facilitate or inhibit tone on a temporary basis. Fast stimulation facilitates tone momentarily by stimulating the antigravity muscles in the neck, trunk, and extremities (McCormack, 1996). It facilitates righting and equilibrium reactions (Trombly, 1983). There is no research that vestibular stimulation has any short- or long-term effect on spasticity (H. Cohen, personal communication, December 18, 1997).

One should avoid neck hyperextension posture during vestibular stimulation of patients with a history of posterior circulation stroke or vertebrobasilar insufficiency. Vestibular stimulation is not indicated in those with Meniere's disease. Nausea and vertigo can result.

Ottenbacher (1983) completed a comprehensive literature review of vestibular stimulation applied to healthy infants, infants at risk, and children with developmental delays. Based on this review, the literature indicated that vestibular stimulation had positive effects on "arousal level, visual exploratory behavior, motor development, and reflex integration" (Ottenbacher, 1983, p. 338).

Practical techniques of effective vestibular stimulation were documented in a study of 38 children who were severely retarded, developmentally delayed, multiply handicapped, and nonambulatory. A suspended car seat was used for upright stimulation, and a suspended hammock was used for supine stimulation. The control group used sensorimotor therapy alone. The experimental group received 13 weeks of vestibular stimulation. The findings revealed that the experimental group achieved statistically significant gains in reflex integration and gross and fine motor skills. It was observed, however, that children without spasticity "made better gross motor and reflex gains than those subjects with spasticity" (Ottenbacher, Short, & Watson, 1981, p. 9).

Electrical stimulation*. NMES is most commonly applied to the antagonistic muscle to stimulate or strengthen that muscle and to inhibit the agonist via reciprocal inhibition (Katz, 1996). Figure 6 depicts a typical usage of electrical stimulation in occupational or physical therapy, facilitating the shoulder abductors (supraspinatus and middle deltoid) and attempting to inhibit the shoulder adductors.

The first author incorporates electrical stimulation with functional activity or uses electrical stimulation to provide the necessary groundwork for functional activity. Therapists may use functional electrical stimulation to facilitate scapular elevation and shoulder scaption to promote independent feeding in a patient with quadriplegia. Therapists may also chose to facilitate the tibialis anterior muscle during gait. A recent study of children with cerebral palsy showed that electrical stimulation strengthened the triceps surae muscle, improving gait and decreasing equinovalgus posture of the foot (Carmick, 1995).

The typical treatment time range for functional electrical stimulation is 10 to 15 min. The literature reviews vary in their reports of duration of therapeutic effect. Katz (1988), in his spasticity literature review, reported a 1-hr therapeutic effect. Doraisamy (1992), on the other hand, reported an effect lasting up to 24 hr.

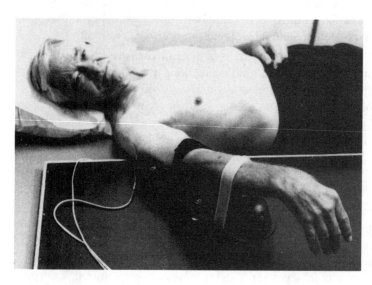

Figure 6. Electrical stimulation facilitating shoulder abduction.

There have been two recent studies using NMES in adults with hemiplegia that challenge commonly held beliefs. The first study demonstrated that electrical stimulation of the agonist failed to produce reciprocal inhibition of the antagonist. NMES was shown to strengthen the extensor digitorum communis muscle in the forearm; however, reciprocal inhibition of the spastic finger flexors did not occur, as assessed by electromyography (Hines, Crago, & Billian, 1993). The second study demonstrated that electric stimulation can result in decreasing spasticity when applied directly to a spastic muscle. This study revealed a reduction in wrist flexion tone with adult patients with stroke. The reduction in tone may be attributed to muscle fatigue or "autogenic inhibition through increased response of the neurotendinous spindle (Golgi tendon organ)" (King, 1996, p. 64). Precautions and contraindications include not using electrical stimulation over a "recent fracture or soft tissue repair (tendon or nerve), on patients with vascular compromise, over demand-type pacemakers, or pregnant women" (Bonzani, 1997, p. 4). Avoid NMES in the cranial or upper cervical region with cerebrovascular accident (CVA), transient ischemic attack, or patients with seizure disorder. Exercise caution when considering NMES/TENS in the cognitively impaired. Adverse skin reactions can occur (Bonzani, 1997). Also this modality should be avoided in patients with cardiac arrhythmia (Giebler, 1990). Pape (1994) precautioned against the liberal use of electrical stimulation in children:

> ...Large eccentric forces may result in sudden injury to tendons or epiphyseal plate and repetitive strain injuries may be produced by periods of forced muscle contracture....NMES must be approached with caution and a full understanding of the potential for the potential for harm as well as benefit. (p. 285)

Table 1 outlines parameters of electrical stimulation devices. It should be mentioned that the settings may differ among different units and manufacturers (Giebler, 1990).

Biofeedback. EMG biofeedback has been used to relax spastic muscles and to facilitate the antagonistic muscles (Swann, van Wieringen, & Fokkema, 1974). It has been shown to improve gait and ameliorate foot drop in patients with stroke (Intiso, Santilli, Grasso, Rossi, & Caruso,1994). Auditory biofeedback has been employed to help improve sitting balance and head control (Giebler, 1990). Biofeedback has not been widely used by clinicians treating spasticity. An extensive review of biofeedback is in Basmajian and DeLuca (1985).

Orthokinetic cuff. The cuff has two parts—an active field and an inactive field. The active field (any elastic bandage) is placed over the

Table 1
Parameters of Electrical Stimulation Devices and Techniques Used to Decrease Spasticity

Devices/Techniques	Pulse Frequency (rate)	Pulse Duration (width)	Intensity, mA
FES NMES	0 to 150 pps	100 to 700 µsec	0 to 100
Low-voltage current	35 pps most common	300 µsec most common	
Medium frequency "Russian" stimulation	1,000 to 100,000 Hz	N/A	0 to 100
	2,500 Hz modulated at 50 bursts per sec most common		
High-voltage pulsed current HVPGS	1 to 120 twin pps	5 to 200 µsec	0 to 2,500
	50 pps most common	20 µsec most common	
High-rate TENS Conventional TENS	40 to 150 pps	20 to 300 µsec	0 to 50
Electroanalgesia	85 pps most common	75 µsec most common	
Low-rate TENS Acupuncture-like TENS	1 to 25 pps	20 to 250 µsec	0 to 100
Electroanalgesia	2 pps most common	220 µsec most common	

Note. TENS = transcutaneous electrical nerve stimulation; FES = functional electrical stimulation; pps = pulses per second; Hz = Hertz, NMES = neuromuscular electrical stimulation; mA = milliamp; HVPGS = High-voltage pulsed galvnic stimulation. From: Giebler, K. B. (1990). Physical modalities. In Glenn & Whyte (Eds.), *The practical management of spasticity in children and adults.* Copyright 1990. Reprinted with permission.

muscle belly of the antagonist. The inactive field is placed on the spastic muscle, providing continuous pressure and decreasing other sensory input. It is made inactive by repeated stretching or sewing to eliminate the elasticity (Giebler, 1990; Trombly, 1983).

Splinting

Splinting plays an important role in the management of spasticity. Splints are used early in the flaccid patient for support and in the mild to moderate spastic patient to maintain a functional position or to help restore ROM. However, there are many controversial factors in splint use.

Many factors need to be taken into consideration when studying the efficacy of spasticity reduction with splinting including splint schedules, splint styles, objective measures of tone, patient satisfaction, and duration of use (Langlois, Pederson, & MacKinnon, 1991).

Spasticity splinting is usually based on Bobaths' principles of reflex inhibiting postures. Patients and caregivers need to be educated in appropriate splint application, wearing schedules, and recognition of early signs of skin breakdown. Orthotics specialists are skilled in bracing and splinting and should be considered members of the health care team. However, even the finest splints can be problematic when used excessively, leading to skin problems or fixed contractures. In particular, the metacarpalphalungral joints are prone to develop irreversible extension contractures.

Upper Extremity Splinting Literature Review

Adult hemiplegia. Langolis, Pederson, and MacKinnon (1991) studied nine adults with hemiplegia with a finger spreader splint and found that spasticity reduced the most in the group wearing the splint 22 hr a day, compared to a 6-hr-a-day wearing schedule and a 12-hr-a-day wearing schedule.

There has been some controversy in the realm of volar versus dorsal splinting in adult hemiplegia. McPherson, Kreimeyer, Aalderks, and Gallagher (1982) studied 10 adults with hemiplegia to determine if dorsal and volar resting splints reduce hypertonus, and if so, what splint was more effective. No significant differences were found when analyzing tone reduction related to dorsal versus volar splints. Rose and Shah (1987) reported that tone was reduced in both dorsal and volar spasticity of wrist flexors on 30 patients with hemiplegia after 2 hr of splint wearing. Their outcome measures included passive ROM and resistance to passive extension.

Cerebral spasticity. Langlois, MacKinnon, and Pederson (1989) completed a comprehensive review of the literature from 1959 to 1989 on the subject of hand splinting and cerebral spasticity. They analyzed dorsal versus volar splinting, finger spreader splints, and cone splints. They noted that clinical observation and some scientific evidence revealed a reduction in hypertonus secondary to splinting. They concluded that "splinting patients with hand dysfunction as a result of spasticity remains a controversial treatment technique because of a paucity of research, methodological weakness in study designs, and contradictory results from investigations" (Langlois, MacKinnon, & Pederson, 1989, p. 113). Clearly, more research is needed.

Cerebral palsy. A single-subject study of a short opponens thumb splint to counteract carpometacarpal adduction improved the child's grip strength, cube stacking, and Box and Blocks test scores in 4 weeks (Goodman & Bazyk, 1991).

Five children with spastic hemiplegic cerebral palsy received benefit from another style of orthosis that controls thumb adduction. A cortical thumb orthosis was developed and deemed effective in all five children, improving a previously ulnar raking type prehension pattern to a radial grasp, using a three-jaw chuck or lateral pinch. Before splinting, the children mostly performed unilateral exploration. However, after splinting they exhibited more bilateral exploration (Currie & Mendiola, 1987).

Hand Splinting: Intrinsic and Extrinsic Factors

It is important to plan your splint choice on the basis of spasticity—intrinsic or extrinsic—and whether patients exhibit both types simultaneously. Extrinsic hand spasticity often masks underlying intrinsic spasticity. Both types can lead to the development of permanent contractures and hygiene problems (Keenan, Todderud, Henderson, & Botte, 1987).

Extrinsic hand spasticity can involve the flexor digitorum sublimis, flexor digtorum profundus, and flexor pollicis longus. Splinting should focus on flexion contracture management of the proximal and distal interphalangeal joints. Some patients respond to individual finger gutter splints, while other patients respond to a spasticity ball splint.

Intrinsic spasticity involves the lumbricals, dorsal interossei, abductor pollicis brevis, flexor pollicis brevis, and opponens pollicis. Chronic intrinsic spasticity can lead to the development of swan-neck deformities. The clinician will expect to find metacarpalphalangeal joint flexion posturing with joints, adduction of the fingers, and abduction and extension of the thumb (Keenan, Todderud, Henderson, & Botte, 1987). The authors have had success managing mild to moderate intrinsic hypertonus with a finger spreader cone-style splint.

Soft palm protector splints are useful for patients with both intrinsic and extrinsic spasticity. When spasticity is severe and positioning cannot be maintained with splinting or casting, the clinician needs to discuss refering the patient to a physiatrist for medical/surgical spasticity management strategies such as nerve blocks, intrathecal baclofen, or orthopedic surgery.

Types of lower extremity splints. The first author has found both the Roylan® Preformed Antispasticity Ball Splint (Figure 7) and the cone-style Roylan® Deluxe Spasticity Hand Splint[4] (Figure 8) useful for patients with flexion tone. Readers are referred to

---

[4] Smith & Nephew, Inc., Rehabilitation Division, One Quality Drive, P.O. Box 1005, Germantown, WI 53002-8205.

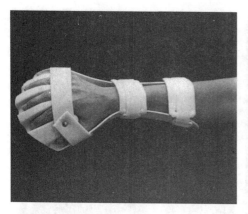

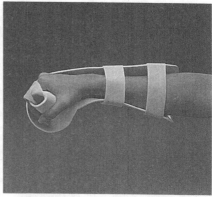

Figure 7. Roylan® preformed antispasticity ball splint. Photograph courtesy of the Rehabilitation Division, Smith & Nephew, Inc.

Figure 8. Roylan® Deluxe spasticity hand splint (cone style). Photograph courtesy of the Rehabilitation Division Smith & Nephew, Inc.

McPherson (1981), Milazzo and Gillen (1998), and Snook (1979) and for additional styles of spasticity reduction splints.

Clinicians can splint in combination with casting. Remember, patients may require a combination of treatment strategies. The following section reviews casting indications and procedures.

Lower extremity casting. The most common lower extremity splint or brace is the ankle–foot orthosis (AFO). It is used to compensate for equinovarus, equinovalgus, "foot drop" (paretic or plegic ankle dorsiflexors), or equinus deformity, on a temporary or permanent basis. AFOs are often fabricated by orthotists.

Ogilvie, a certified orthotist, finds progressive AFOs very useful in the rehabilitation of patients with stroke. Progressive AFOs are used early in the patient's rehabilitation with the goals of permitting early ambulation, preventing equinovarus deformities, and providing proprioceptive input to the affected lower extremity. Figure 9A depicts a progressive AFO. This AFO is fabricated using a high temperature thermoplastic elastomer. A tone-inhibiting footplate is incorporated into the orthosis along with high dorsal trimlines to allow maximum midfoot and hindfoot control. Ankle joints are also molded into the orthosis, but are maintained in a locked position until the patient's hip and knee control improve. When adequate hip and knee control are achieved, the ankle joint is released into free dorsiflexion with a 90° plantarflexion stop (Figure 9B). The dorsal foot trimlines are adjusted to allow only what support is needed over the midfoot and hindfoot.

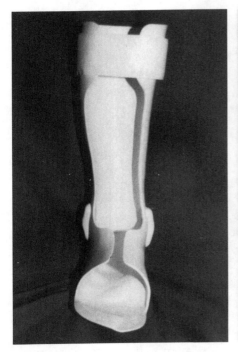

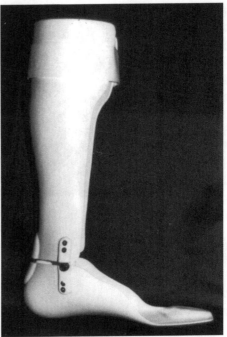

Figure 9A. Anterior view of progressive ankle–foot orthosis (AFO). Note dorsal trimlines that control the midfoot and hindfoot. Designed by Garry Ogilvie, Certified Orthotist.

Figure 9B. Lateral view of progressive ankle–foot orthosis (AFO) that has been articulated with a 90° plantar stop. Note that the dorsal trimlines have been lowered to decrease midfoot and hindfoot control. Designed by Garry Ogilvie, Certified Orthotist.

Another noteworthy lower extremity splint is the toe spreader splint. A Bandaid® Moleskin and hard cell foam splint was invented by Utley and Thomas. This splint inhibits flexion and adduction of the toes. For commercially available lower-extremity splints, please refer to the Resource section.

Casting

The positive effect of casting on spasticity and contractures in the upper extremities has been well documented in the literature (Booth, Doyle, & Montgomery, 1983; Cherry & Weigaand, 1981; Feldman, 1990; King, 1982). Casting in inhibitive postures has been shown to be effective in tone reduction (Cruickshank & O'Neill, 1990; Hill, 1994; Yasukawa, 1990). Casting is believed to inhibit the excitability of gamma and alpha motor neurons. Maintained pressure, neutral warmth, and constant position of a joint with static lengthening of a muscle may also contribute to its efficacy (Hylton, 1990). Katz (1988) noted significant decreases in both dynamic and static reflex sensitivity with casting.

Serial casting is indicated when an extremity has moderate severe hypertonus and is at risk for becoming contracted. Typical diagnoses that may warrant casting include traumatic brain injury, CVA, and cerebral palsy. Occasionally casting is indicated for persons with spinal cord injury. Special cautions include the following (Patricia Neal Rehabilitation Center Policy and Procedure Manual, 1998): (a) avoid casting patients with sensory loss,[5] (b) do not serial cast over unhealed fractures (Hylton, 1990); (c) avoid casting highly agitated or confused patients who may inflict harm on themselves or others with their casts; and (d) avoid casting over open wounds—however, it may be feasible to cut a window in a cast to permit wound care (Robison, 1997). Sometimes properly padded casts are used to treat poorly healing wounds. Resistant wounds in the sensitive feet of diabetics or persons with leprosy are sometimes treated with casting. A walking cast can be fabricated to eliminate pressure over the sore by transferring forces to other areas of the foot. Avoid any other medical complication deemed to be a contraindication by the physician.

Casts can be made of plaster or fiberglass, solid or bivalved (bivalved casts, in actuality, are considered splints). Serial casting involves the application of a solid cast and changing it every 3 to 7 days. The primary author uses fiberglass more often due to its lightweight nature, durability, and soil-resistance. Plaster casts are indicated in patients who are fearful of the cast saw, as they can be soaked off. Plaster casting tape is less expensive than fiberglass, however it is more time consuming in application and maintaining the correct position of the joint while casting and in drying time (P. Cannon, personal communication, July 11, 1998). Appendix H shows different types of upper and lower extremity casts.

Occupational and physical therapists at Patricia Neal Rehabilitation Center (PNRC) list the following materials needed for solid cast fabrication:

1. Cast saw
2. Plastic basin or bucket

---

[5] Occasionally, physicians will order casting on patients with sensory loss. It is recommended to monitor these patients very closely and remove casts every 1 to 2 days until skin tolerance is determined. A positional cast splint (bivalved cast) can be removed every 30 min to 2 hr if skin tolerance is extremely poor (P. Cannon, personal communication, June 11, 1998). In the hands of an experienced therapist, these patients can indeed be casted.

3. Cast spreaders

4. Plastic-covered, blunt-end scissors

5. Surgical gloves (for fiberglass casting only)

6. Gowns (protect patient and therapist's clothing)

7. Masks and goggles (needed for cast removal)

8. Cotton cast padding (for fiberglass cast)

9. Orthopedic felt padding (for plaster cast)

10. Cotton tubular stockinette—2 in, 3 in., or 4 in.

11. 1/16-in. sticky-backed foam (pad bony prominences)

12. Casting tape—fiberglass or plaster casting tape—2 in, 3 in., or 4 in.

Additional materials needed for bivalve casting:

1. Adhesive tape or Bandaid® Moleskin

2. Ace wrap or Velcro® straps

Before casting, the occupational and physical therapists need to have in-service or continuing education training, or both. It is strongly recommended that therapists inexperienced in casting seek supervision and assistance from experienced therapists.

Casting should commence only after receiving a written physician's order. The therapist and physician should discuss the need for X rays or bone scan to rule out heterotopic ossification before casting (Hylton, 1990). At times, diagnostic blocks are preformed before casting. Long-term blocks such as phenol or botulinum toxin–type A are indicated to reduce or obliterate spasticity, thus easing the casting process. Refer to chapter 4 for more information on nerve blocks.

Procedure for fiberglass cast application at PNRC.

1. Objectively assess and document ROM and muscle tone.

2. Apply stockinette to the extremity without wrinkles, allowing enough material to fold back over the cast at both ends. Slit stockinette at joint bends to overlap—this prevents wrinkles (e.g., at cubital fossa of elbow when extension lacks 80° or more.

3. Position the body part to be casted at resting range, not with excessive stretch. The extremity to be casted is then stretched to about 5° less than maximum ROM.

4. Pad all bony prominences or areas deemed likely to develop pressure areas with 1/16-in. foam or felt. Avoid pressure or extra material build-up on areas that have superficial nerves. The therapist can shape the felt in a donut around areas like elbows or heels.

5. Apply rolls of padding in a spiral manner, overlapping one-half width of the padding. Use more narrow widths for distal parts, and more wide widths for proximal parts. Usually apply two to three layers of padding—to include enough padding above and below level of cast to be folded back into the cast. Keep in mind that excessive padding can decrease inhibition.

6. Therapists need to don surgical gloves before fiberglass casting or chafing will occur with skin contact. Dip fiberglass tape in tepid water and hold for 5 to 8 sec, three times. Then squeeze out excess water gently without wrinkling the material.

7. Apply fiberglass[6] in a spiral manner beginning about 1/4 in. to 1/2 in. below the starting and ending points of the padding, overlapping width of the fiberglass. It is very important that the first layer of fiberglass is not wrinkled next to the patient's skin. Check for weak spots and reinforce them accordingly. Be careful not to wrap fiberglass too tightly, especially at the ends of the cast, as this may cause swelling. Avoid indenting the cast. Fiberglass dries quickly, so it must be applied swiftly. The cast will warm and may even get hot while it dries. It will dry within 30 min to 1 hr.

8. Fold edges of stockinette and padding over the cast borders. This serves to pad the sharp edges of the fiberglass and thus protects the patient's skin. The edges of the cast must be flared, not rolled. Flaring means the therapist places their fingers inside the ends of the cast and trying to spread it slightly to prevent a bottleneck effect that can cause edema. Remember, spastic muscles do contract and one must allow extra room for that contraction so the cast does not tighten and cause edema or pressure areas. Secure folded stockinette to cast with final roll of fiberglass.

9. Check for skin color as well as color of nail beds during and after casting. After casting, always check for (a) red areas, especially at cast edges; (b) difference in temperature between casted and uncasted extremity; (c) pulses at distal points to

---

[6] The fiberglass package should be squeezed before opening to check for suitability for application. The roll should feel pliable and soft. Do not use tape that feels hard. In addition, fiberglass begins to interact and harden when the package is open and exposed to the air. With each roll of fiberglass, you have about 1 min to complete wrapping. Fiberglass will stick to clothing and leave a permanent residue (P. Cannon, personal communication, June 11, 1998).

the cast; (d) complaint of pain;[7] or paresthesia; (e) excessive swelling; (f) dusky veins; and (g) discoloration of hand or foot. Observe the color of the patient's nailbeds. If they appear bluish in color this could indicate poor capillary refill.

Procedure for plaster cast application at PNRC. Refer to the above fiberglass casting procedure. The differences are as follows:

1. Dip plaster in tepid water, holding the end free for about 10 sec until thoroughly moistened and pasty. Squeeze out excess water without wringing the roll of plaster.

2. Apply three to five layers of plaster in a spiral manner, using the same technique as with fiberglass. Avoid indenting or pulling the plaster. The plaster warms as it begins to dry. Read the package of plaster casting tape to determine length of drying time, as there is variation 2 to 24 hr.

3. Hint: Therapists will need to discard the plaster or water bucket in a designated area, not a regular sink. Plaster will completely wash out of clothing.

Bivalve preparation for splint wear.

1. Check inside of cast for rough edges through padding material. If there are rough edges, remove padding and try to smooth with other plaster or file down with a file or cast saw, especially with fiberglass. Replace padding.

2. Take away and add padding as indicated.

3. Tape edges of padding and stockinette around cast edges. Moleskin® or foam can be used if necessary. Three-inch adhesive tape is usually sufficient and more cost-effective.

4. Apply to patient and secure with Ace® wrap or Velcro® straps. Ace® wrap is almost always required. Velcro® straps aid the caregivers in cast application. Pull ace wrap tightly to remove elasticity, otherwise the cast halves can shift, pinching the patient's skin and causing blood blisters and skin breakdown.

---

[7] Patients may complain of pain, even though the cast may appear to be applied correctly. This pain is usually related to stretching. Do not remove the cast immediately, however, do continue to monitor tolerance. Occasionally intense stretching may cause "storming" of low-level, acute brain injury patients. These patients can manifest physiological changes, including sweating, increased blood pressure, and agitation. In these cases, the patient may need to be recasted with less of a stretch with more frequent cast changes. These patients may be a candidate for positional casting (bivalved as opposed to solid).

5. Check fit, make sure no pinching is occurring.

6. Devise wearing schedule. Usually start with 2 hr on and 2 hr off, progressing to 4 hr on and 2 hr off. The wearing schedule should be more conservative if the patient's skin tolerance is low. The schedule should be posted where it is easily visible for caregivers. Skin checks are recommended every 2 hr initially. The ultimate goal is building up the patient's tolerance to withstanding all night wear.

Potential bivalve splint problems include swelling secondary to decreased circulation or cast weight, skin pinching where the bivalved cast comes together, and pressure areas due to wrinkles or rough edges.

Procedure for cast removal at PNRC.

1. Draw cutting lines on the sides of the cast so that it may be cut into anterior and posterior halves. It is helpful to make the posterior half of the cast larger, so the extremity will fit in it like a gutter.

2. Cut cast with cast saw into anterior and posterior halves. Try not to make the cuts across a joint or muscle belly if the cast is to be used as a splint, this can increase the risk of pressure areas or skin problems. The "in and out" saw method is recommended, as cast saws cut by vibration. If the cast is padded appropriately, do not be over-fearful of cutting the patient. Patients will often complain of discomfort, and this is usually due to vibration. If the patient feels heat, remove saw immediately.

3. Spread the halves with the cast spreader. The cast will spread with ease, if it is cut all the way through. If it does not spread easily, insert cast saw in uncut areas and re-saw. If a plaster cast is not completely dry, it will crumble.

4. Cut padding (on at least one side) with blunt-end scissors. If cast is to be used as a splint, both sides of the padding must be cut.

5. Lift one half of the cast open, lift out extremity carefully.

6. Document postcast ROM measurements and objective tone assessments.

7. Perform passive ROM, and, if possible, active ROM of joint before another cast is applied.

8. The extremity should be cleaned with an alcohol rub between casts (Hylton, 1990). Do not wash or apply lotion to the extremity because the moisture can be trapped in the next cast and cause skin breakdown.

9. Check skin for swelling and pressure areas or skin breakdown. If a pressure area is found, therapist can window the next cast, bivalve next cast, or wait until the pressure area heals.

10. The first cast should be removed after 1 to 3 days for a skin check. Subsequent serial casts can be changed weekly or more often if deemed necessary.

When to discontinue serial casting. Serial casting should cease when the desired position is achieved and tone is manageable. If there is no evidence of increased passive ROM after two to three casts are removed, casting must cease. Closer monitoring, decreasing wearing time, or applying a different style of cast may be indicated if problems arise with casting or splints. Casting may be resumed when deemed necessary (P. Cannon, personal communication, June 11, 1998).

Drop-out casts. Drop-out casts have a portion of the cast removed (dropped out) to expose part of the extremity. One must not cut out too much of the cast or the positional hold will be lost. This permits ROM in the desired, limited range but prevents movement in the direction of the hypertonus. Elbow or wrist drop-out casts are an effective way to work on active joint ROM while it is casted. Gravity can also assist in increasing ROM. A common style of drop-out cast is the elbow drop-out cast. The goal is to gain elbow extension while preventing undesired elbow flexion. Using NMES on the triceps while wearing a drop-out cast can facilitate active movement (Figure 10). Other modalities or facilitation techniques can be applied as appropriate. Drop-out casts are removed, and the patient is re-casted when significant increases in ROM have occurred or if the cast has become ineffective.

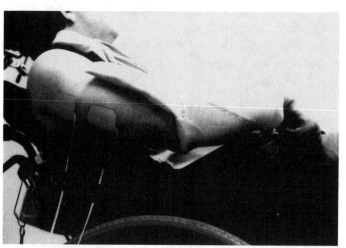

Figure 10. Elbow drop-out cast with electrical stimulation facilitating the triceps. (See Appendix H for illustrations of upper extremity casts).

Review Questions

1. Using the Modified Ashworth scale, spasticity would be rated ___ if there is a marked increase in muscle tone throughout most of the ROM.

2. Using Trombly and Scott's 3-step spasticity scale, spasticity would be rated ___ if the stretch reflex occurred in the middle of the range.

3. Which of the four traditional therapeutic theoretical approaches focuses on the facilitation of normal movement patterns using spiral and diagonal movement components?

4. List three facilitation techniques that stimulate the primary afferent nerve of the muscle spindle.

5. What are the contraindications to superficial heat application on patients with spasticity?

6. How does ultrasound relax a spastic muscle?

7. Electric stimulation is *most commonly* placed over the spastic agonist to reduce tone, true or false?

8. Dorsal splinting has been shown to be more effective than volar splinting on adults with hemiplegia, true or false?

9. When serial casting, list the symptoms or signs that may occur if the cast is too tight.

10. Air splints are considered to be an inhibitive treatment, true or false?

Chapter 3
Review of Current Oral and Intrathecal Medications

Oral medications are used to temper spasticity. Unfortunately, oral medications act systemically rather than in the specific areas of concern, and the doses needed to control spasticity are often too high to be tolerated by the patient. It is helpful to the physician to have feedback from the occupational or physical therapist as to the benefits, lack thereof, or side effects noted when new medications are added. The therapist's overall impressions of spasticity reduction, as well as objective spasticity assessments and timed functional tasks are useful in treatment evaluation.

Therapists need to be aware of adverse effects of these medications, as some of these effects can influence the patient's ability to participate in therapy. Table 2 outlines the six most commonly prescribed medications in spasticity management. According to Katz (1996), baclofen is the drug of choice for spinal spasticity and dantrolene sodium is the drug of choice for cerebral spasticity.

Intrathecal Baclofen
Indications

Intrathecal baclofen involves the surgical implantation of a baclofen delivery pump into a patient's abdomen with an attached catheter connected to the lumbar intrathecal space. Patients with chronic, severe, disabling spasticity are considered candidates for intrathecal baclofen. These patients have not responded adequately to oral medication or traditional spasticity reduction techniques. Diagnoses that may benefit from intrathecal baclofen include spinal cord injury, cerebral lesions including cerebral palsy, and multiple sclerosis (Lazorthes, Sallerin-Caute, Verdie, Bastide, & Carillo, 1990). Occupational and physical therapists will encounter possible candidates for

Table 2
Oral Medications

Medication	Mechanism of Action (MOA)	Indications	Common Adverse Reactions	Selected Warnings
Baclofen USP Lioresal[a]	Exact MOA not completely known. Inhibits mono- and polysynaptic reflexes at the spinal level. Also has supraspinal action.	First line for spinal spasticity and MS. Especially useful for painful flexor spasms. The efficacy in stroke, CP, and Parkinson's disease has not been established.	Drowsiness, dizziness, weakness, fatigue, confusion, nausea, urinary symptoms, insomnia	Abrupt withdrawal can produce seizures and hallucinations. Poor tolerance noted after stroke.
Dantrolene Sodium Dantrium®[b]	Produces skeletal muscle relaxation by interfering with calcium release within the muscle and dissociates the excitation–contraction coupling.	First line for cerebral spasticity (i.e., stroke, CP). Also used in all upper motor neuron disorders such as MS and SCI.	Drowsiness, dizziness, weakness, malaise, fatigue, diarrhea, abdominal pain	Symptomatic hepatitis—fatal and nonfatal, active hepatic disease, avoid driving when first used.
Tizanidine HCl Zanaflex®[f]	Reduces spasticity via increasing presynaptic inhibition of motor neurons. An agonist of alpha-2 adrenergic receptor sites.	Reduces spasticity in MS and SCI.	Dry mouth, somnolence, weakness, dizziness	Hypotension, elevation of liver function tests, sedation, visual hallucinations
Diazepam Valium®[c]	Exact MOA not completely known. Inhibits mono- and polysynaptic reflexes at the spinal level. Also has supraspinal action on thalamus, hypothalamus, and limbic system.	Reduces UMN spasticity	Drowsiness, fatigue, ataxia at higher doses	Abrupt withdrawal can produce seizures, avoid driving, physiological and psychological addiction possible.
Clonidine Catapres®[d]	Reduces sympathetic outflow from CNS, decreases heart rate and blood pressure	Labeled as antihypertensive. Also reduces spasticity, used primarily in SCI	Dry mouth, drowsiness, constipation, dizziness, sedation	Hypotension; however, abrupt withdrawal can result in nervousness, agitation, headache, and a rapid rise in blood pressure that can cause a rare hypertensive CVA.

Table 2 (cont.)
Oral Medications

Medication	Mechanism of Action (MOA)	Indications	Common Adverse Reactions	Selected Warnings
Chlorazepate dipotassium Tranxene®e	Probably similar to diazepam. Depressant effect on the CNS.	Labeled for anxiety management and adjunctive therapy for seizure management. Also reduces spasticity.	Drowsiness, complaints dry mouth, fatigue, ataxia, dizziness, nervousness	Physiological and psychological dependence, same as diazepam

Note. Information on Lioresal®, Dantrium®, Valium®, Catapres, and Tranxene are derived from Goodman & Gilman's *The pharmacological basis of therapeutics* (1995). Zanaflex® is newly approved in the United States, as of January 1997. The information about Zanaflex® was obtained from the *Physicians Desk Reference* (1998).

a Novartis, 59 Route 10, East Hanover, NJ 07932

b Proctor and Gamble Pharmaceuticals, Inc., P.O. Box 368, Ridgefield, CT 60064

c Roche Products, Inc., Manati, Puerto Rico.

d Boehringer Ingelheim Pharmaceuticals, Inc., 900 Ridgebury Road, P.O. Box 368, Ridgefield, CT 06877-0368

e Abbott Laboratories, 100 Abbott Park Road, Abbott Park, IL 60064

f Athena Neurosciences, Inc., 800 Gateway Blvd., South San Francisco, CA 94080.

CNS = central nervous system; CVA = cerebrovascular accident; CP = cerebral palsy; MS = multiple sclerosis; SCI = spinal cord injury.

intrathecal baclofen in hospitals, outpatient clinics, home health care, and extended care facilities. The pump has also been used with patients with spinal cord injury who have severe episodic muscle spasms (Abel & Smith, 1994). Intrathecal baclofen can help patients who have been using inappropriate medications to relieve chronic pain or sleep pattern disturbances secondary to severe spasticity (Savoy & Gianino, 1993). It can also help patients with severe spasticity in many muscle groups, when it would not be practical to provide numerous injections of phenol or botulinum toxin (Glenn & Elovic, 1997). In 1996, intrathecal baclofen was approved by the Food and Drug Administration (FDA) for use in brain injury. It is recommended that patients with traumatic brain injury (TBI) wait at least 1 year before trying intrathecal baclofen therapy, allowing for spontaneous neurological recovery. However, for patients with TBI with severe spasticity, intrathecal baclofen should be implanted much earlier to prevent the development of contractures. For spinal cord injury, Medicare recommends a minimum of 6 weeks of noninvasive treatment before an intrathecal baclofen trial (J. Leahy, personal communication, July 1998).

A smaller pump, 10 cc, (SynchroMed®) is used in children. The safety of intrathecal baclofen in children under the age of 4 has not been established (Blumenkopf, 1997).

The primary benefit of intrathecal baclofen is that it is a fully reversible, nondestructive procedure. Often it is considered before permanent procedures such as orthopedic surgery or neurosurgery (Siegfried, Jacobson, & Chabal, 1992).

Oral Versus Intrathecal Baclofen

Oral baclofen is distributed equally into the brain and spinal cord, and it has difficulty penetrating the blood–brain barrier (Lazorthes et al., 1990). Intrathecal baclofen permits effective cerebrospinal fluid concentrations to be achieved with resultant plasma concentrations 100 times less than those occurring with oral administration (*Physicians Desk Reference*, 1997). Therefore, considerably lower drug doses can be used with intrathecal administration (Blumenkopf, 1997). It has been estimated that oral medications are ineffective in approximately 30% of patients with severe spinal spasticity. Intrathecal baclofen is delivered directly into the cerebral spinal fluid, which is the site of action for effective reduction of spasticity. The centrally mediated side effects of drowsiness and confusion associated with oral baclofen are rarely seen in intrathecal delivery (Savoy & Gianino, 1993).

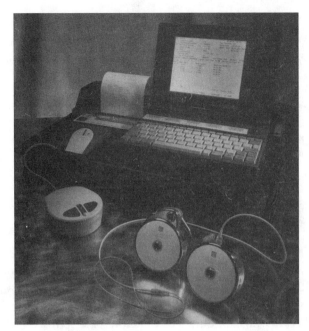

Figure 11. The SynchroMed® intrathecal baclofen system: computer, hand-held telemetry, programmer pump, and catheter.

Mechanism of Action

The exact mechanism of intrathecal baclofen as an antispasticity drug is not completely understood. Baclofen is believed to be a structural analog of the inhibitory neurotransmitter gamma-aminobutyric acid (GABA), and may exert its effects by stimulation of the GABA's receptor subtype. Thus it may increase inhibition of neurons that in turn would be excitatory of primary alpha motor neurons innervating skeletal muscle (Hardman & Limbird, 1995).

Types of Pumps

Three manufacturers of intrathecal baclofen delivery pumps have been described in the literature. The SynchroMed®[8] infusion system supplied by Medtronic Company, Inc. is widely used in this country. It is programmable via computer telemetry and has the ability to adjust dosages to meet individual needs. For example, a patient may need more medication at night to relieve painful night spasms and less in the day when spasticity can be used for transfers (Savoy & Gianino, 1993). The SynchroMed® pump was approved in 1992 by the FDA to treat severe debilitating spasticity (Rawlins, 1995). Refer to Figure 11 for depiction of the SynchroMed® system. In June, 1996,

---

[8] Medtronic, Inc., Neurological Division, 800 53rd Avenue, NE, Minneapolis, MN 55421.

37

the Medtronic pediatric pump was approved (Blumenkopf, 1997). The Arrow International Model 3000[9] pump (also used for cancer chemotherapy) is indicated when continuous infusion of baclofen is needed, such as when through prior experience of that patient with pumps, the dose needed for control of spasticity is fixed. The authors recommend that constant infusion pumps not be used first, because frequent dose change cannot be easily achieved with a fixed dose infusion pump. In the United Kingdom and Europe, the Cordis Secor[10] pump is available. It is manufactured by Cordis in Valborne, France. It is a manually operated pump, implanted close to the skin, where the patient palpates the buttons. Intentional overdose is possible with this pump. There are risks of infection and skin necrosis with this pump (Gardner et al., 1995).

Procedure for Implantation of the SynchroMed® Pump

Prior to scheduling the test dose, patients need to have spasticity increasing factors ruled out—such as urinary tract infection or fecal impaction. Before implantation, patients are given a test bolus of intrathecal baclofen via lumbar puncture or a spinal catheter (*Physicians Desk Reference*, 1997). The test bolus of baclofen is administered by a neurologist or a neurosurgeon. A placebo bolus may also be administered to rule out any possible placebo effect (Blumenkopf, 1997). Patients are deemed candidates for pump implantation if they maintain a 2-point reduction in their Ashworth score or spasm score for 4 hr after the test bolus (Abel & Smith, 1994). It may take up to a month for significant tone reduction in the upper extremities.

The pump can be implanted percutaneously under local anesthesia or under general anesthesia contingent on patient or surgeon preference as well as the degree of spontaneous muscle spasms present (Lazorthes et al., 1990). The patient is positioned in side-lying and an incision is made in the left abdominal wall, placing the pump in a subcutaneous pocket (Abel & Smith, 1994). The subcutaneous catheter is placed into the lumbar subarachnoid space with a Tuohy needle and advanced to the level of T-12 (Abel & Smith, 1994). A medtronic pump catheter has been implanted as high as T-6 (J. Leahy, personal communication, November, 1998). The catheter is then subcutaneously tunneled to the left abdominal wall and connected to the pump (Abel & Smith, 1994). The pump is externally programmed through a radio-frequency-linked telemetry wand connected to a computer (Abel & Smith, 1994). Spinal X rays help confirm correct

---

[9] Arrow International, 1600 Providence Highway, Walpole, MA 02081

[10] Cordis, Valbonne, France.

catheter position and can detect kinks and disconnections. Special overexposed X rays can detect malfunctions in the pump rotor (Gianino, 1993).

Contraindications

There are several types of patients for whom this treatment is not appropriate. Patients with major impairment of renal, hepatitic, or gastrointestinal function; pregnancy; history of epilepsy; or hypersensitivity to baclofen should not undergo a test bolus. The patients who do not experience a reduction in spasticity of the maximum 100-µg. test dose are not candidates for intrathecal baclofen therapy. Conversely, patients whose spasticity reduced too much are not candidates (Abel & Smith, 1994). If the test dose eliminated spasticity that was needed in upper and lower extremities to perform activities of daily living (ADL), these patients were not considered candidates for treatment (Lazorthes et al., 1990).

Onset and Duration

The onset occurs 30 min to 1 hr after the test bolus. A peak effect of baclofen occurs at 4 hr after dosing and the effects last 4 to 8 hr (*Physicians Desk Reference*, 1997).

Adverse Effects

Complications can result from intrathecal baclofen and some are potentially fatal. These risks are reduced when intrathecal baclofen is provided by a competent and experienced team (Gardner et al., 1995). Occupational therapists must be aware of the potential adverse effects and report suspicious symptoms and signs to the patient's physician.

Complications can be categorized in three ways: technical, infectious, or pharmacological. Technical problems can include a leaking pump or malfunctioning pump. A device pumping too much medication can cause baclofen overdose; signs include respiratory depression and coma (Lazorthes et al., 1990). Catheter malfunctions can include kinks, breaks, or disconnections (Abel & Smith, 1994). The SynchroMed® will beep if it needs to be refilled or if a new battery is needed (Gianino, 1993).

Local infection around the subcutaneously implanted pump has been documented (Lazorthes et al., 1990). Temporary chemical noninfectious meningitis can result from intrathecal drug delivery.

The top five pharmacological side effects according to a study of 150 patients on maintenance doses include: (a) hypotonia, (b) somnolence, (c) headache, (d) convulsion, and (e) urinary retention

(*Physicians Desk Reference*, 1997). Other side effects may include feeling light-headed, slurred speech, nausea, itching, and double or blurred vision (Gianino, 1993). Acute withdrawal of intrathecal baclofen can result in hallucinations (*Physicians Desk Reference*, 1997). Siegfried, Jacobson, and Chabal (1992) reported that patients with spinal cord injury with quadriplegia experienced disorientation, seizures, and intermittent loss of consciousness after abrupt cessation of intrathecal baclofen.

Drug Tolerance

Patients can develop a physiological tolerance to intrathecal baclofen, usually within the first year. After the first year, no significant changes in dosage were detected in a study of 18 patients with spinal cord injury who were treated with intrathecal baclofen (Akman, Loubser, Donovan, O'Neill, & Rossi, 1993). A baclofen holiday is recommended for 2 to 8 weeks if tolerance occurs, and morphine can be used during this time (Gianino, 1993).

Efficacy

Intrathecal baclofen's indications for spasticity management in patients with multiple sclerosis and spinal cord injury have been well documented in the literature (Abel & Smith, 1994; Becker et al., 1995). Lazorthes and colleagues (1990) found intrathecal baclofen to be beneficial in reducing spasticity in individual cases of spinal ischemia, transverse myelitis, and cerebral palsy and in an ischemic cerebral lesion. Further evidence of its efficacy in children with cerebral palsy has been documented in a randomized double-blind placebo-controlled study (Albright, Cervi, & Singletary, 1991). Gerszen, Albright, and Johnstone (1998) have shown that intratheal baclofen reduced the need for lower-extremity orthopedic surgery.

Cost

The estimated combined cost of the surgery and the Medtronic SynchroMed® pump is around $18,000 to $25,000. Mark-up and hospital costs vary. Follow-up, maintenance costs, and refills (4 to 12 times per year) may average $3,660 per year (J. Leahy, personal communication, November 1998).

Occupational and Physical Therapy After Implantation

Occupational and physical therapy may resume 1 month after implantation (M. Barry, personal communication, June, 1998).

Review Questions

1. List four of the six common oral medications used for spasticity management.

2. What is the only oral medication known to exert its mechanism of action at the skeletal muscle level?

3. What spasticity medication has a chemical structure similar to the neurotransmitter GABA and is considered to be the drug of choice for spinal spasticity?

4. What oral spasticity medication is also used to lower blood pressure and reduce sympathetic outflow from the central nervous system?

5. All of the oral antispasticity medications cause sedation, true or false?

6. What is the treatment of choice for generalized, severe spasticity not responding to oral medication?

7. Contrast the use of oral versus intrathecal baclofen.

8. What types of patients are not considered appropriate for intrathecal baclofen?

9. What are the three major potential complications in intrathecal baclofen drug delivery?

10. How often is a baclofen pump refilled? Describe the implantation procedure.

Chapter 4

Review of Nerve Blocks in the Treatment of Spasticity: Functional Implications in Occupational and Physical Therapy

Nerve blocks involve the introduction of a chemical agent via injection to a nerve (or motor point) to impair its function either on a short- or long-term basis. Nerve blocks are administered by physicians specializing in anesthesiology, neurology, orthopedic surgery, or physiatrics. Not all of the above-mentioned physician specialists perform blocks. The therapist will need to discuss this matter with the physician specialist. There are short-acting and long-acting nerve blocks. Short-acting drugs are primarily used for diagnostic purposes. Long-acting blocks are used to temporarily weaken the spastic agonist (Katz, 1996). Both short- and long-acting blocks will be discussed. The authors hope the readers will be able to refer appropriate candidates for nerve blocks upon completion of this section.

It is important to understand the difference between fixed or static deformities versus dynamic deformities. Fixed deformities may include any of the following: soft tissue contracture of muscle and ligament, capsular contracture, joint deformity with bony block, bridging of bone between two bones that normally move in relation to each other, or heterotopic ossification. Some soft tissue types of fixed deformities can be remedied by serial casting, however some other types of soft-tissue contractures and all bony contractures require orthopedic surgery. Dynamic deformities are caused by the unilateral pull of spasticity. When the spasticity is reduced with (a) a combination of inhibitive techniques to the spastic agonist and facilitation techniques to the antagonist or (b) nerve blocks, or both, full range of motion (ROM) is restored.

Short-Term Blocks

There are three primary purposes for the administration of short-term, diagnostic blocks. First, diagnostic blocks can temporarily eliminate pain and muscle tone so that dynamic contractures or static contractures can be differentiated (Keenan, 1987). Second, diagnostic blocks can assess the potential effect of a longer acting block (Katz, 1996). Third, they can oppress the spastic muscle so that strength and control of the antagonistic muscle groups can be evaluated (Keenan, 1987).

The diagnostic block procedure is the same as percutaneous phenol block, except different chemical agents are used. Please refer to section on *Procedure for percutaneous phenol motor point blocks* later in this chapter for procedure details.

Mechanism of Action

Katz (1996) described the mechanism of action of local blocks, such as lidocaine, as: "temporarily block conduction by interfering with the increase in permeability of the sodium ions that normally occur when the membrane is depolarized" (p. 597). Table 3 gives a list of chemical agents and length of effect for diagnostic blocks (Keenan, 1981). Table 4 provides information of common sites for diagnostic blocks.

The second author occasionally opts to administer epinephrine (Adrenaline) with the diagnostic blocking agent. Epinephrine serves to constrict blood vessels and confine the anesthetic agent to a local area for longer lasting effect. Side effects from epinephrine can include tachycardia, elevated blood pressure, anxiety, and fear (Hardman & Limbird, 1995).

Table 3
Short-Term Blocks: Chemical Agents and Length of Effect

Agent	Duration
Procaine (Novacaine®)[a]	>1 hr
Lidocaine (Xylocaine®)[b]	1 to 2 hr
Bupivacaine (Marcaine®)[c]	7 hr

Note. [a] Novocaine®, Sanofi Winthrop, 90 Park Avenue, New York, NY 10016. [b] Xylocaine®, Astra Pharmaceutical Products, Inc., 50 Otis Street, Westborough, MA 01581. [c] Marcaine® Abbott Laboratories, 1 Abbott Park Road, Abbott Park, IL 60064-3500.

Table 4
Diagnostic Blocks—Common Sites and Goals

Site	Goals
Brachial plexus	Obliterate tone and pain in the entire upper extremity
Musculocutaneous nerve	Diminish biceps tone, enabling evaluation of the strength and tone of triceps
Median nerve at elbow	Evaluate flexion deformity of the wrist and fingers
Median nerve at carpal canal	Evaluate role of median nerve innervated muscles in a thumb adduction deformity
Ulnar nerve at Guyon's canal	Determine role of intrinsic spasticity, which is often masked by extrinsic spasticity
Sciatic nerve	Diminish hamstring spasticity and evaluate knee extension range
Femoral nerve	Eliminate quadriceps tone and evaluate knee flexion range
Obturator nerve	Diminish spasticity of hip adductors, and evaluate hip abduction, standing balance, and gait
Posterior tibial nerve	Eliminate tone in posterior calf muscles that can cause a hindfoot equinovarus deformity

Diagnostic blocks are a relatively inexpensive procedure. The cost range is $95 to $300 depending on the area treated and the practitioner's geographic location (R. Chironna, personal communication, December, 1998).

Clinical Vignette

The authors recently evaluated a patient who was 15 months post-traumatic brain injury and incomplete cervical six spinal cord injury. He had restricted active elbow flexion of 0 to 90° and passive 0 to 100°. This restriction impeded his ability to actively or passively touch his face. A diagnostic block was administered for the following reasons: (a) to obliterate triceps spasticity, thus permitting assessment of biceps function, (b) to rule out the presence of myostatic contracture, and (c) to determine the potential effect of a long-term block. The second author administered a diagnostic block of 0.5% bupivacaine and 2.0% Xylocaine to the motor points of the long (Figure 12) and lateral heads of the triceps. The patient's active ROM improved to 110° and passive improved to 130° 5 min after the block was completed. It was now possible for the patient to passively touch his face (Figure 13). It was felt that the patient would benefit from a long-acting block and daily occupational therapy to strengthen the antagonists, the elbow flexors.

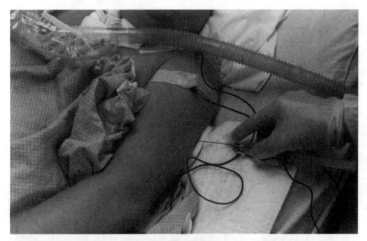

Figure 12.
Diagnostic block: long head of the triceps. Needle is connected to a nerve stimulator which aids in the localization of the motor points of the radial nerve.

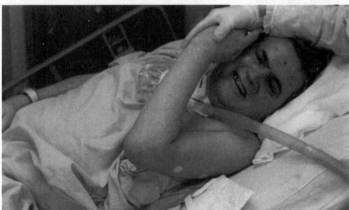

Figure 13.
Functional gain after block to lateral and long heads of the triceps: The patient is able to passively touch his head.

Long-Term Blocks

Candidates

Occupational therapists will encounter candidates for long-term blocks in skilled nursing units, rehabilitation centers, hospitals, outpatient facilities, and home health care. The following is a general candidate list for patients with acquired spasticity that holds true regardless of the type of long-term block:

1. Patients with acquired spasticity, during the period of neurological recovery (Botte, Abrams, & Bodine-Fowler, 1995; Keenan, Tomas, Stone, & Gersten, 1990)[11]

---

[11] The typical period of spontaneous neurological motor recovery for a stroke patient is 6 months; for a patient with traumatic brain injury, 18 months (Botte, Abrams, & Bodine-Fowler, 1995).

2. Patients who have severe spasticity in one group of muscles masking the potential of the weak antagonistic muscles (Roper, 1987)

3. Patients with moderate to severe spasticity that is causing a dynamic deformity, where it is believed that without intervention the dynamic deformity will lead to a fixed deformity

4. Patients who are unable to maintain satisfactory ROM with use of traditional occupational and physical therapy techniques. These techniques are often very time consuming (Charles, 1997)

5. Patients with spasticity that interferes with nursing care, hygiene, functional movement (Glenn & Whyte, 1990), and positioning (Wilson, 1992)

6. Patients whose spasticity causes such severe pain that they are not able to participate in therapy (Wilson, 1992)

7. Patients who are unable to tolerate bracing secondary to spasticity

The following list discusses long-term block candidates for children with cerebral palsy:

1. Children with cerebral palsy to manage severe spasticity in order to tolerate a manual stretching program until they are old enough to participate in rehabilitation protocols for orthopedic surgery (Hisey & Keenan, 1999)

2. Children with cerebral palsy participating in muscle reeducation (M. Weinstein, personal communication, December 8, 1997)

Contraindications

There are three general contraindications for long-term nerve blocks. Patients with fixed joint deformities are generally not candidates for nerve blocks. An exception to this situation may be a patient with both static and dynamic deformity in which it is believed serial casting may ameliorate the fixed deformity, and the block would temper the dynamic deformity. Patients who are allergic to the chemical agents proposed and patients who benefit from their spasticity are not candidates for nerve blocks. Please refer to the phenol and botulinum sections for contraindications specific to each agent.

Four common types of long acting nerve blocks will be profiled: percutaneous phenol motor point, closed branch phenol, open branch phenol, and botulinum toxin-A. Each block will be discussed in terms of indications, procedure of administration, onset, duration, and efficacy. The three types of phenol blocks will be listed according to degree of invasiveness, progressing from the least invasive to the most invasive.

Phenol Blocks

Phenol can be characterized as *neurolytic*, meaning actual destruction of the axon cell membranes, myelin, or the motor end plate (Hisey & Keenan, 1999). Ethyl alcohol has been used in the same manner as phenol, but it has not been widely used as it offers no superior benefit over phenol (Katz, 1996).

Phenol affects the nerve through two mechanisms of action. First it has a short-term anesthetic effect on the nerve (Greenbaum, Young, & Frank, 1993). Second, phenol denatures the protein in a peripheral nerve, causing axonal degeneration and demyelination of the nerve. In large nerves, phenol acts on the axons in the peripheral portion of the nerve, not influencing the central fibers (Glenn & Elovic, 1997). "The axon then regenerates because the continuity of the nerve sheath has not been disrupted" (Keenan, 1987, p. 65). This regeneration occurs when the axons reach their respective motor end plates and motor function thus returns (Botte et al., 1995).

Percutaneous phenol motor point block. Motor point blocks are used to decrease spasticity stemming from nerves that are deep and difficult to reach via direct injection. This type of block is also used for mixed nerves by attempting to hit the motor points and thus avoiding sensory fibers that can cause painful paresthesias. Motor point blocks are used when the desired result is to reduce spasticity, not to completely eliminate it. Table 5 lists common sites for percutaneous phenol blocks.

Procedure for percutaneous phenol motor point blocks. The patient is positioned either side-lying or recumbent, depending on the area to be injected. Xylocaine is often used as a local anesthetic (Hecht, 1992). Children may benefit from the application of a local anesthetic cream, such as Emla®[12] cream. Emla cream is applied 45 min before injection. A motor point block is performed by direct injection of phenol into muscles, with the injection directed specifically to motor points within the muscle. The motor points within a muscle are thought to be areas either where the motor nerve branches course through the muscle or areas where there is a high concentration of motor end plates (Botte et al., 1995). A Teflon®-coated needle is connected to an electrical stimulator, and a syringe of phenol is attached to the hub (Hecht, 1992). The motor points are located with the electrical stimulator. The physician knows that a motor point is

---

[12] Emla® cream, Astra USA Inc. West Borough, MA 01581.

Table 5
Percutaneous Phenol Blocks-Common Sites and Goals

Site	Goals
Pectoralis major	Reduce shoulder adduction and internal rotation tone
Biceps and/or brachioradialis[a]	Decrease elbow flexion tone
Pronator teres	Reduce forearm pronation tone
Palmaris longus FCU, and/or FCR	Decrease wrist flexion tone
Flexor digitorum sublimis	Reduce finger flexion tone, especially the PIP joints
Flexor digitorum profundus	Reduce finger flexion tone, especially the DIP joints
Thenar eminence	Decrease median nerve driven thumb intrinsic spasticity
Adductor brevis	Reduce hip adductor tone
Posterior tibialis	Decrease plantar flexion and hindfoot varus

Note. FCU = Flexor carpi ulnaris; FCR = flexor carpi radialis; PIP = proximal interphalangeal; DIP = distal interphalangeal.

[a] Dynamic electromyography (EMG) of the brachioradialis has shown to exhibit severe, continuous spasticity in stroke and traumatic brain injured patients (Keenan et al., 1993). If the patient has difficulty obtaining the last 30° of elbow extension, the therapist may suggest a motor point block to the brachioradialis. When physicians inject the brachioradialis, they must be careful to avoid injection of the extensor carpi radialis longus and brevis or an undesirable loss of wrist extension may occur.

located when a maximum contraction is elicited with minimal electrical stimulation; for example, if a biceps brachii motor point was stimulated, the elbow would flex (Botte & Keenan, 1988). The physician will also know if a sensory branch is inadvertently stimulated as the patient will verbally or nonverbally respond to pain. Sometimes the muscles are located via electromyography (EMG) instead of a nerve stimulator. The physician often refers to an EMG localization guidebook, such as Geiringer's *Anatomic Localization for Needle Electromyography*, and aims for the large concentration of motor points (usually in the midpoint of the muscle). The motor end plate is detected by listening for the "end plate noise," or uninhibited firing of motor units. Spastic muscles sound loud on EMG. Once the physician locates the desired motor point, aspiration is performed to rule out vascular puncture, which would be very dangerous.

The aqueous phenol is then injected into the motor point. To avoid excessive edema, the physician should not inject more than five motor points in one region (e.g., forearm) (Keenan, 1987). An ice bag is applied to the injected limb, and elevation is recommended.

Onset and duration. Motor point injections either take immediate effect or take effect within the first 24 hr (Botte & Keenan, 1988). They average around 2 months, which is a shorter duration than a closed motor branch block or a surgical block. Again, spasticity is reduced with percutaneous blocks, not eliminated.

Efficacy of percutaneous phenol motor point injections. Four studies involving efficacy of percutaneous motor point injections will be highlighted. Keenan et al. (1990) found motor point injections of the biceps and brachialis muscle lasted as long and were equally effective when compared with surgical phenol injection in 17 adults with brain injury. Botte and Keenan (1988) found that percutaneous phenol blocks to pectoralis major reduced spasticity for patients with traumatic brain injury and stroke. Garland, Lilling, and Keenan (1984) documented an average gain of 30° of active wrist extension after percutaneous motor point blocks were administered in the wrist flexors. Chironna and Hecht (1990) documented gains in external rotation after motor point injection to the subscapularis muscle, the primary muscle responsible for internal rotation of the shoulder.

It is important to note that the spastic subscapularis is often mislabeled as adhesive capsulitis (frozen shoulder) in the adult patient with spastic hemiplegia or hemiparesis. The second author has noted that these patients rarely ever develop adhesive capsulitis. The shoulder is "frozen" or rendered immobile as a result of the spastic subscapularis. If this is not recognized, and the alleged frozen shoulder is treated under manipulation, a fractured humerus can result.

Closed motor branch phenol block. Closed motor branch block is indicated in nerves that have easily identifiable motor branches. This type of block can turn upper motor neuron spasticity into lower motor neuron flaccidity for weeks or months.

Contraindications of this type of block include avoiding mixed nerves (nerves in which the sensory and motor components run together) because the loss of sensation is undesirable. If a sensory nerve is inadvertently injected, the patient can develop painful causalgia (Glenn, 1990). Please refer to Table 6 for a listing of common sites for closed motor branch blocks (Botte et al., 1995).

Closed motor branch procedure. The procedure is similar to the motor point block procedure except a nerve stimulator is used to locate the motor branch; that is, the axon, not the motor point. The physician knows that the motor branch is located when the nerve is stimulated enough to cause a contraction or desired motion in the spastic muscle with minimal current. One injection to the motor branch is sufficient.

Onset and duration. The onset of clinical effect is the same as it is in percutaneous phenol blocks, occurring immediately or within the first 24 hr. The duration varies from 4 to 6 months.

Efficacy. Hecht (1992) demonstrated increased external rotation, flexion, and abduction of the shoulder following closed motor branch

Table 6
Closed Motor Branch Phenol Blocks—Common Sites and Goals

Site	Goals
Upper and lower subscapular nerves	Diminish tone in subscapularis, thus decreasing internal rotation spasticity that impedes normal external rotation PROM
Recurrent branch of median nerve	Diminish tone in abductor pollicis brevis, flexor pollicis brevis, and opponens pollicis
Musculocutaneous nerve	Diminish biceps tone
Obturator nerve	Diminish hip adduction tone
Lumbar paraspinal nerve	Reduce hip flexion tone
Tibial nerve at popliteal fossa	Reduce spasticity in all ankle plantar flexors

Note. PROM = Passive range of motion.

block of the injection of the subscapular nerve in 13 adult patients with hemiplegia. The authors have noted on many occasions that adults with hemiplegia who are undergoing the subscapular block experience extended spasticity reduction in their entire upper extremity. The authors believe this supports the belief and experience of neurodevelopmental (NDT) practitioners that spasticity reduction in proximal musculature can indeed promote spasticity reduction in distal musculature.

One study had shown few side effects and positive results with closed motor branch blocks to the musculocutaneous nerve, even though it contains both motor and sensory nerves (Botte et al., 1995). Another study by Wassef (1993) noted a reduction in hip adductors in patients with paraplegia and multiple sclerosis via closed motor branch blocks of the obturator nerve. This treatment facilitated nursing care in the bedridden patients and improved gait in the patients with multiple sclerosis.

Cost. The estimated cost of percutaneous and closed motor branch phenol blocks including the medication and procedure is $359 (R. Chironna, personal communication, November 25, 1998). This is far less costly than botulinum toxin-type A.

Open motor branch block. Open motor branch phenol blocks are not administered as often as they were 5 years ago, owing to the advent of botulinum toxin. Open motor branch blocks are also known as a surgically isolated motor branch blocks. Although this procedure is seldom performed, there are five situations in which open phenol blocks may be desirable:

1. When complete paralysis of a spastic muscle is desired (Keenan, Todderud, Henderson, & Botte, 1997)

2. When the desired nerve cannot be safely reached by way of closed motor branch block

3. When an unsatisfactory result has occurred with percutaneous blocks, as may be in the case of percutaneous hip adductors (obturator nerve motor points) or the median nerve innervated muscles of the thenar eminence (Keenan, 1987)

4. When multiple surgical procedures are being performed on the hand and the final muscle balance is uncertain" (Keenan et al., 1987, p. 735)

5. When providing long-term tone management in patients with anoxic brain trauma, as their neurological recovery is slow (M.A.E. Keenan, personal communication, September, 1998)

Common sites include the ulnar nerve at Guyan's canal, the posterior tibial nerve, the femoral nerve, and the obturator nerve.

Open motor branch block procedure. Open motor branch blocks are performed by surgeons (Braddom, 1996). The patient is anesthetized. The skin and muscles are dissected, and the motor branch is isolated and confirmed with the use of a nerve stimulator. The surrounding tissues are protected from phenol with a saline-moistened gauze. The block is completed when a 1-cm segment of a nerve is translucent and electrical stimulation does not produce a motor response (Keenan, Todderod, Henderson, & Botte, 1987).

Onset and duration. The onset of effect is immediate, and the typical duration is 2 to 8 months (Botte et al., 1995).

Efficacy of open motor branch blocks. Keenan, Todderud, Henderson, and Botte (1987) found a reduction in intrinsic tone in all 21 hands after open motor branch phenol blocks. Because phenol is a temporary neuroblative technique, 13 (62%) of the hands had a return of spasticity after 6 months. Eight hands had slight or no return of spasticity as a result of neurological recovery.

Moore and Anderson (1991) reported effective reduction of spasticity in the posterior calf muscles in nine patients with head and spinal cord injuries. The motor branches of the tibial nerve were injected in 16 limbs. Moore and Anderson believed that this procedure helped prevent the development of equinovarus contractures of the foot and ankle. This procedure enabled five patients who were nonambulatory before the block to become ambulatory. Petrillo and Knoploch's (1988) study of 59 patients found that administering open tibial nerve blocks reduced spasticity in all patients, with the average reduction of tone lasting 28.7 months.

Cost. The cost of an open branch phenol block varies depending on the duration and complexity of the procedure as well as the physician's geographic location. An estimated surgeon's fee is $1,000 (M. A. E. Keenan, personal communication, November 25, 1998).

Side effects of phenol. The most common side effects include bleeding, edema (Wilson, 1992), weakness for the first few hours or days (Katz, 1996), and transient soreness at the injection site. If a sensory nerve is inadvertently injected, dysesthesia and burning paresthesias may occur (Glenn & Whyte, 1990). Less common side effects include: (a) allergy to phenol, (b) pneumothorax, (c) neuritis (Chironna & Hecht, 1990), (d) compartment syndrome (Wilson, 1992), (e) scarring and fibrosis of surrounding structures (Young, 1994), (f) local infection, and (g) deep vein thrombosis (Glenn & Whyte, 1990).

Contraindications to phenol. Pierson, Katz, and Tarsy (1996) wrote that phenol is relatively contraindicated in anticoagulated patients. Chironna, Glass, and the second author disagree with this statement. These physicians have performed more than 300 phenol blocks with a large percentage of these patients being anticoagulated. No serious complications were experienced. These physicians believe phenol blocks are safe and effective when administered by experienced physicians in normal anticoagulated patients with an international normalized ratio of 2.0 to 3.0, and the patient's anticoagulant is withheld 48 to 12 hr before the block (S. Glass & R. Chironna, personal communication, September 17, 1997).

Pre- and Postphenol Block Occupational and Physical Therapy

Evaluation and treatment. Physicians and therapists alike will find pre- and postblock therapy evaluations very valuable in assessing the efficacy of the block. ROM measurements, both active and passive, of the muscles affected by the block are indicated, and an objective scale to quantify spasticity, like the Modified Ashworth Scale, is needed. Refer to Chapter 2 for details of evaluation test items. Postphenol block occupational or physical therapy evaluation should take place 24 hr after injection. Therapists must report paresthesia or causalgia to the physician who administered the block. This problem is usually handled in one of three ways: (a) The physician may order high-rate transcutaneous electrical nerve stimulation (TENS) (with a rate setting 85 pps, width 75-sec) to manage the pain until spontaneous pain resolution has occurred (Glenn & Whyte, 1990); (b) oral medications such as tricyclic antidepressants, nonsteroidal anti-inflammatories, or steroids may be used to decrease pain, and are most often needed for 1 to 3 weeks (Glenn & Elvoic, 1997); or (c) the phenol block may be repeated.

The physician may order anti-inflammatory medication to ameliorate postblock soreness. Therapists need to treat edema with compressive wraps, icing, and elevation.

Muscle reeducation of the antagonist should begin immediately at a frequency of three times per week for 4 weeks and reevaluate. The use of functional electrical stimulation to the antagonist is often indicated. Electrical stimulation will increase the strength of the muscle and decrease the tendency of that muscle to fatigue (Botte et al., 1995). The therapist may consider providing the patient with a home electrical stimulation unit. Therapists must not be too zealous with stretching a muscle in which the tone has rapidly been reduced, as sprains and strains can result (Glenn & Elovic, 1997).

If the phenol block is administered with the goal of easing care giving in a nonfunctional extremity when it is believed that reducing tone will not improve function, the postblock therapy treatment is different. The patient should only be seen for home exercise program training and possibly splinting.

The authors have noted a low incidence of motor point injections having no effect. When this happens, a repeat block is performed a few days later and usually the desired effect is achieved.

Using phenol blocks in children with cerebral palsy. Physicians are divided over the issue of using phenol blocks in children. Some physicians feel phenol blocks should be a standard part of pediatric care. Yadav, Singh, U., Dureja, Singh, K., and Chaturvedi (1994) noted a reduction in spasticity in 116 children with spastic cerebral palsy in whom ambulation and perineal care was effective. The block reduced spasticity in all cases, 11 blocks of which were repeated secondary to the first block not having a therapeutic effect. The blocks allowed bracing in some of the children who were previously unable to wear a brace. Yadav et al. (1994) believed their results should warrant more widespread use of phenol in children with spastic cerebral palsy.

A few physicians have written that phenol is not indicated in cerebral palsy, claiming there is not the typical "recovery phase" as there is in cerebrovascular accident (CVA), incomplete spinal cord injury, and traumatic brain injury (Botte et al., 1995). Furthermore the toxic dosage of phenol is not known in the pediatric population. Morrison, Matthews, Washington, Fennessey, and Harrison (1991) noticed an increased incidence in cardiac arrhythmia in pediatric cerebral palsy patients who were anesthetized with halothane and who were receiving motor point phenol injections. They recommended electrocardiogram monitoring regardless of the type of general anesthesia used with phenol blocks. With the advent of EMK® cream, general anesthesia is often not needed.

Short acting diagnostic blocks are typically preferred over phenol blocks in cerebral palsy when planning orthopedic surgery, because the duration of the block is 7 hr or less.

Botulinum Toxin-Type A

Botulinum toxin-type A is commonly referred to by its trade name Botox®. There are seven other types of botulinum toxin. The other types are being developed and are not yet approved by the FDA. Botulinum toxin-type A is actually a toxic protein produced by the anaerobic bacteria *clostridium botulinum* (Borg-Stein, Pine, Miller, & Brin, 1993). Although this bacteria produces the disease of botulism and is considered one of the most potent poisons known to man, it is a beneficial medication for nerve blocks.

Mechanism of action. Botulinum toxin-type A (hereafter referred to as botulinum toxin) can be described as chemodenervating, which means an interruption of the normal chemical exchange on a receptor level. Botulinum toxin exerts its effect at the neuromuscular junction by inhibiting the release of acetylcholine, thus causing a flaccid paralysis when the muscle receives no further chemical stimulation (Borg-Stein et al., 1993).

Indications. Botulinum toxin has been approved by Medicare to aid in the treatment of the following conditions: (a) strabismus, (b) blepharospasm, (c) multiple sclerosis, (d) spastic hemiplegia, (e) infantile cerebral palsy, and (f) torticollis. It has been used to block spasticity in patients with traumatic brain injuries. Botulinum toxin has also been used to treat craft dystonias such as musician's cramp and writer's cramp (Charles, 1997). The FDA has approved botulinum toxin usage for blepharospasm, strabismus, and hemifacial spasm of the 7th cranial nerve (Allergan Medical Information Line, 1-800-433-8871).

Candidates for receiving botulinum toxin injections are generally the same as for phenol. Refer to the long-acting nerve block indication section in this chapter. Botulinum toxin does have one main advantage over phenol. This advantage is that there is no chance of unwanted sensory side effects; for example, burning paresthesia. For this reason it is often selected over phenol in smaller distal limb

---

[13] Allergan Pharmaceuticals, Inc., 2525 Dupont Drive, PO Box 19534, Irvine, CA 92713-9534.

musculature where there are mixed sensory-motor nerves (Pierson, Katz, & Tarsy, 1996).

Clinical Vignette

Figure 14 depicts a patient with a hemiplegic hand with painful, severe spasticity as a result of a stroke. The patient had no active movement distal to her forearm before botulinum toxin injections. The injections were administered with the following goals in mind: (a) to open up her hand, thus decreasing pain and easing hygiene, and (b) to reveal any potential movement in her hand that may have been masked by severe spasticity. Botulinum toxin was injected in the following muscles: flexor digitorum profundus, flexor digitorum sublimis, first and second lumbricals, flexor pollicis longus, and palmaris longus. Two weeks later, the same patient was photographed in sitting (Figure 15). Her finger flexor tone was rated flaccid. In standing (Figure 16), her finger flexor tone was rated mild. Wrist flexion tone was rated moderate in both at rest and antigravity positions, as the primary wrist flexors were not injected. The goals of pain reduction and easing hygiene were met. The patient now has a 40° arc of combined wrist flexion or extension, and a 20° arc of thumb metacarpalphalangeal flexion or extension.

Cost. The wholesale cost of Botulinum toxin as of May 1998, was $352.14 per 100 unit vial. It may take 3 to 6 vials per adult patient, depending on the size of the area and number of muscles to be injected (Charles, 1997; Gooch & Sandell, 1996).

Procedure. There is a strict storage and reconstitutional procedure for botulinum toxin. It is stored in powder form at negative 5°C. It is diluted before use in preservative-free normal saline (Caine, 1993). Children may benefit from the application of a local anesthetic

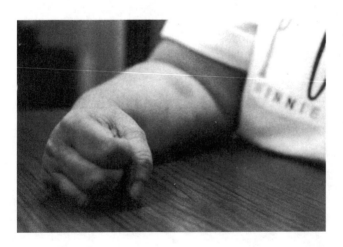

Figure 14. Spastic hemiplegic hand. Note presence of both intrinsic and extrinsic spasticity.

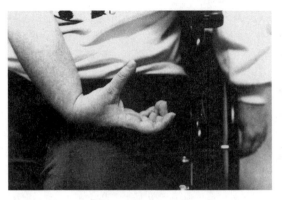
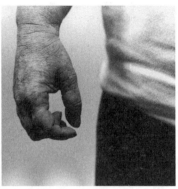

Figure 15. Reduction of spasticity (sitting position) after botulinum toxin injections.

Figure 16. Reduction of spasticity (antigravity position) after botulinum toxin injections.

cream, such as Emla® cream, to numb the injection site. Emla® cream is applied 45 min before injection, and Tegaderm[14] tape covers the area so children cannot rub the cream off (J. Simpson, personal communication, August 25, 1998).

There are three injection methods. The method chosen may depend on physician preference and the location of the desired muscle. The first method involves using an EMG machine, and no electrical stimulation is given. Using an EMG-guided Teflon® needle, the proper site for intramuscular injection at the motor point is found. The motor end plate noise identifies the site of injection, and recruitment identifies it as being in the correct muscle (Charles, 1997). This method is particularly advantageous when injecting small or deep musculature (Borg-Stein et al., 1993). A second method is known as the "aim and shoot" method. The physician aims for the middle of the muscle, aspirates, then injects. The third method involves the same localization technique as the percutaneous motor point phenol block and uses electrical stimulation (Glenn & Elovic, 1997). A local injectable anesthetic is not used for any of these methods (Katz, 1996). Ice is typically applied after the block. Compressive wraps may be used to reduce edema.

Onset and duration The onset occurs in about 72 hr (Charles, 1997). There are conflicting reports in the literature regarding the occurrence of peak effect. Simpson et al. (1996) reported peak effect occurred between 2 to 6 weeks postinjection. Hesse et al. (1994) reported

---

[14] Tegaderm, 3-M Health Care, St. Paul, MN 55144-1000.

peak effect at 2 to 4 weeks. It has a duration of 3 to 5 months. A patient may require three to four injections per year (Charles, 1997).

Side effects. The most commonly seen side effects of botulinum toxin are very mild. They include local pain, ecchymosis (Grazko, Polo, & Jabbari, 1995), and edema. Edema can be treated with a compression glove or suitable wrap (Yablon, Agana, Ivanhoe, & Boake, 1996). Side effects generally last 1 to 2 days (Koman, Mooney, Smith, Goodman, & Mulvaney, 1994). Dangerous generalized weakness could potentially occur when large doses are used in infants. Less common side effects include undesired weakness, transient fatigue, nausea, and headache (Glenn & Elovic, 1991).

Precautions. Botulinum toxin should not be used during pregnancy or during lactation. It is not indicated in patients who have disorders of neuromuscular transmission such as myasthenia gravis, Eaton-Lambert syndrome, or motor neuron disease (Charles, 1997).

Nonresponse. There are some persons who are immune to botulinum toxin and will not respond to the injection. Other patients may form antibodies after several injections, thus not responding to further injections. This can be evaluated by blood testing. Other reasons for nonresponse may include inadequate dosage, faulty injection technique, improper storage or reconstitution of the toxin, and evolving disease process (Charles, 1997).

Efficacy of botulinum toxin. Nine patients with multiple sclerosis were injected in the leg adductor musculature in a double-blind, placebo-controlled cross-over study. The results showed a significant reduction of spasticity and an ease in perineal care (Snow et al., 1990). Caine (1993) also found a statistically significant reduction of spasticity, measured by the Modified Ashworth Scale, and increased ease of hygiene and a decrease in the frequency of muscle spasm.

The authors' literature search revealed only one article that documented occupational therapy treatment after botulinum toxin injection. The article chronicled a patient with right hemiparesis resulting from a traumatic brain injury (20 years postinsult). She presented with flexed fingers and wrist. Her forearm, wrist, and finger flexors were injected. She was treated in occupational therapy at a frequency of twice weekly for 2 months. The physician's goals of injection were "to reduce spasticity and stretch out (the patient's) arm through serial casting and night-time positioning" (Joe, 1996, p. 317). The patient presented with a flaccid wrist and hand for 2 weeks. The therapist splinted the patient her first day of therapy. A few days later a cast was applied that was to be worn on top of the splint. The patient wore this cast for 1 week. Ring splints were provided to enable the patient to perform activities of daily living (ADL). The patient's home program included ROM, weight bearing, strengthening, and 15 min of daily electrical stimulation to her wrist and finger extensors. The end result was positive. She was able to perform the following activities that she was unable to do before the injection: (a) able to write in clear bold letters, (b) operate a meat slicer with her right hand, and (c) able to pick up utensils with her right hand. The duration of effect was not included (Joe, 1996).

Yablon et al. (1996) injected the wrist flexors in 21 patients with traumatic brain injury, 12 chronic and 9 acute. In the chronic group, active wrist extension improved by a mean of 36.2°, and passive ROM increased 15° to 75° in 11 out the 12 patients. In the acute group, active wrist extension improved by a mean of 42.9°, and passive ROM increased 30 to 100° in 8 out of 9 patients.

Botulinum toxin is also being used in children with spastic cerebral palsy. In a double-blind, placebo-controlled study, 12 children were injected (6 placebo, 6 botulinum toxin). All children were injected in the medial and lateral gastrocnemius muscle, and those with equinovarus were also injected in the posterior tibialis muscle. Five out of six children showed improvement versus two out of six who received the placebo (Koman et al., 1994).

Koman, Mooney, Smith, Goodman, and Mulvaney (1993) treated 27 spastic cerebral palsy children with dynamic deformities with botulinum toxin. The children in group one (*n* = 3) were injected in the paraspinal musculature. The outcome was a decrease in paraspinal spasticity, which eased positioning and permitted the children to rest more comfortably. The children in group two (*n* = 8) were injected in various sites in the lower extremities. All 8 children experienced a reduction in spasticity and improved positioning. Group three included 16 ambulatory children, 10 had equinovarus, and 6 had equinovalgus. All patients experienced an improved gait.

Gooch and Sandell (1996) reported a case study to promote left-sided function in a boy 3 years of age with hemiparetic cerebral palsy. He had flexion posturing of his elbow and wrist and did not have use of his arm. Botulinum toxin was injected in his biceps brachii, brachioradialis, and flexor carpi radialis (FCR). His Ashworth Scale spasticity score in his elbow flexors decreased by 2. Four months later, the effects of the injection waned.

The authors found one case study particularity intriguing. Gooch and Sandell (1996) reported a case of a girl 11 years of age with athetoid cerebral palsy who underwent Botox injection with a goal of relieving severe left hip pain related to chronic movement around her hip. The patient had a history of multiple orthopedic hip surgeries as well as unsuccessful trials of oral medications of dantrolene sodium and baclofen. The iliopsoas, rectus femoris, gluteus medius, and gluteus maximus were injected. One week after the injection, she experienced a dramatic decrease in pain and diminished movements around her hip.

There have been several studies demonstrating the efficacy of botulinum toxin in adults with hemiplegia. Hesse et al. (1994) showed a reduction in spasticity in 11 out of 12 patients with chronic stroke with equinus posturing after injection of the soleus, tibialis posterior, and both heads of the gastrocnemius. Eight out of 12 had improved gait. The effects waned in 8 weeks. Simpson et al. (1996) performed a double-blind placebo-controlled study of 39 patients with chronic stroke. This study showed a significant reduction of upper-extremity flexion spasticity in the biceps brachii, FCR, and flexor carpi ulnaris (FCU) after botulinum toxin injection. Curiously, the patient's grip strength increased, suggesting this neurolytic agent may have reduced tone enough in one set of muscles to "unmask function in a nearby set" (Simpson et al., 1996). It is felt that further long-term studies need to be done in the treatment of spasticity and the cost-effectiveness of botulinum toxin.

Seventeen patients with chronic hemiplegia with severely spastic, nonfunctional upper extremities were injected in the biceps, forearm finger flexors, and FCU. Hand hygiene improved in 14 out of 17 (Bhakta, Cozens, Bamford, & Chamberlain, 1996). Similar results were found in 6 patients with hemiplegia with biceps brachii, FCU, and flexor digitorum profundus injected (Das & Park, 1989).

In the future, other types of botulinum toxin will be released. Whether their effects will be similar to botulinum toxin-type A remains to be seen.

Occupational and physical therapy evaluation and treatment. The therapist should perform an objective spasticity evaluation before the injection and include suggestions on which muscles should be injected. The occupational therapy evaluation should be scheduled 2 weeks postinjection, as this often is the beginning of the toxin's peak effect. Reevaluation is suggested 4 weeks postinjection for those patients who have a delayed onset of peak effect to document changes in function. Contingent on the amount of toxin injected and patient response, the therapist can expect a weakened spastic muscle or a totally flaccid muscle.

Occupational and physical therapy treatment postbotulinum toxin is basically the same as in phenol including muscle reeducation techniques supplemented with electrical stimulation to the antagonist. Splinting and casting will be much easier. Therapy is scheduled three times per week for 4 weeks, then the need for continued therapy is determined on reevaluation. As with phenol, if the block was performed with the goal of reducing tone to ease care giving and improve hygiene in a nonfunctional extremity, regularly scheduled therapy sessions are not needed. One or two sessions may be needed for home exercise training or splinting. A therapist should expect a shorter duration of effect with botulinum toxin (duration 3 to 5 months) when compared to closed motor branch or open motor branch phenol blocks.

Comparison of Phenol and Botulinum Toxin

Phenol has several advantages when compared to botulinum toxin: phenol is less expensive, open and closed motor branch phenol last longer than botulinum toxin, one cannot form antibodies to phenol, and the onset of clinical effect is seen much sooner with phenol— within 24 hr (Botte & Keenan, 1988) as opposed to 2 to 4 weeks (Hesse et al. 1994).

Botulinum toxin has several advantages over phenol. It is an easier procedure to perform since electrical stimulation is often required. There is no chance of undesired sensory side effects (i.e., paresthesia causalgia). For this reason, botulinum toxin is often selected in lieu of phenol in smaller, distal limb musculature where there are vast numbers of mixed nerves (Pierson et al., 1996). Botulinum toxin can be performed without anesthesia (local or general) in children and adults (Koman et al., 1993). The duration of effect is more definitive with botulinum toxin (3–5 months) than phenol (2–8 months). Botulinum toxin wears off rapidly whereas phenol wears off gradually. There is no chance of residual scarring (M.A.E. Keenan, personal communication, September 2, 1998). Patients who have experienced both botulinum toxin and phenol injection report to the authors that botulinum toxin hurts less as it is injected. Refer to Table 7 for a succinct comparison of phenol and botulinum toxin.

Table 7
Comparison of Phenol and Botulinum Toxin-Type A

Characteristic	Phenol-Percutaneous	Botulinum Toxin
Injection location and procedure	Best for larger muscles, especially those with spare sensory innervation	Preferred in smaller, distal musculature where there are vast numbers of mixed nerves
	Physician locates motor point or motor branches with a nerve stimulator	Easier injection technique than phenol
	Emla® cream may be used or local anesthetic injection	Physicians aim for the muscle belly and inject
		At times, EMG muscle localization is needed
		Emla® cream may be used
Mechanism of action	Neurolytic: (a) short-term anesthetic effect on the nerve (b) denatures protein in the nerve demyelination and/or axonal- degeneration occu	Chemodenervating inhibits the release of acetylcholine at the neuromuscular junction
Onset	Immediate or within 24 hr	Initial signs of paresis are within 72 hr Peak effect 2 to 4 weeks
OT/PT postblock evaluation	Schedule 24 hr after block	Initial signs of paresis are within 72 hr Peak effect 2 to 4 weeks
Duration of block	Motor point: 2 to 5 months Motor branch: 2 to 8 months	3 to 5 months
Waning	Gradual	Rapid
Common side effects	Edema at injection site, ecchymosis, local pain	Same as phenol
Less common side effects and complications	Paresthesia, scarring, and fibrosis of surrounding structures	Fatigue, nausea, headache, generalized weakness, infection

Table 7 (cont.)
Comparison of Phenol and Botulinum Toxin-Type A

Characteristic	Phenol-Percutaneous	Botulinum Toxin
Contraindications	Areas where there are high concentrations of sensory nerves, allergy to phenol	Disorders of neuromuscular transmission, such as Myasthenia gravis or Eaton-Lambert Syndrome, or motor neuron disease
Antibody formation	Not possible	Possible, and renders the injection ineffective
Cost of the agent	Negligible	$352.14 per 100 unit vial
		May take 3 to 6 vials per adult patient

Note. OT = occupational therapy; PT = physical therapy.

Review Questions

1. Contrast the use of short- versus long-term blocks.

2. What are the differences between a fixed (static) versus a dynamic joint deformity?

3. When is a short-term block indicated?

4. How can long-term blocks facilitate the achievement of therapy goals?

5. What are the contraindications to long-term blocks?

6. A girl 6 years of age has "thumb-in-palm" deformity. She has weak movement in her thumb extensors. What type of nerve block would you recommend? To what muscles?

7. A man 40 years of age recovering from a traumatic head injury has spasticity in his elbow flexors, impeding full elbow extension –30 to 150°. What type of nerve block would you recommend? What muscle would you recommend?

8. What type of spastic muscle deformity is often mislabeled adhesive capsulitis in the patient with spastic hemiplegia? How is this treated properly?

9. How soon after a phenol block would you schedule a therapy evaluation? After a botulinum toxin injection?

10. What percent chance postphenol block is there of a patient to experience paresthesia? What is the chance (%) after postphenol block that the patient will experience paresthesia? How is paresthesia treated by the doctor and by the therapist?

11. What treatment modalities would one select after a long-term block to the wrist flexors? What new goals can be addressed after the block?

12. If a patient did not respond to a long-term block, what would you do?

13. The typical period of neurological motor recovery for a stroke patient is _____ months.

14. For a patient with traumatic brain injury, the period is _____ months.

Chapter 5
Orthopedic Surgery in the Treatment of Spasticity: Implications in Occupational and Physical Therapy

O ccupational and physical therapists will encounter clients who can benefit from surgical intervention to manage spasticity. The following discussion will highlight two common scenarios where orthopedic surgery is beneficial—for patients manifesting decreased functional standing or walking tolerance secondary to equinovarus deformity and for patients enduring painful contractures of the hands, elbows, and shoulders.

Patients with spastic cerebral palsy, traumatic brain injury, or stroke may experience decreased standing or walking tolerance due to equinovarus deformity (Figure 17). The surgical procedure of split anterior tibialis tendon transfer (SPLATT) (Figure 18) accompanied by Achilles tendon lengthening can ameliorate this deformity and aid in the development of a more functional gait with better active dorsiflexion and eversion.

Orthopedic surgery candidates also include residents in extended care facilities or recipients of home health care manifesting painful hands, elbows, or

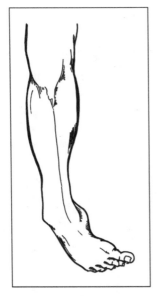

Figure 17. Equinovarus deformity. From M. A. E. Keenan, S. H. Kozin, & A. C. Berlet (Eds.). (1993). *Manual of orthopaedic surgery for spasticity* (p. 97). New York: Raven Press, Ltd. Reprinted with permission.

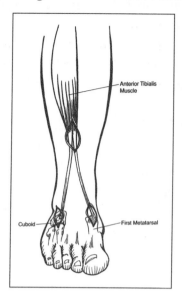

Figure 18. Completed split anterior tibialis transfer (SPLATT). From M. A. E. Keenan, S. H. Kozin, & A. C. Berlet (Eds.). (1993). *Manual of orthopaedic surgery for spasticity* (p. 103). New York: Raven Press, Ltd. Reprinted with permission.

shoulder contractures. The severity of these contractures may render maintenance of basic hygiene virtually impossible. Such patients traditionally have not tolerated splint-wearing well due to their high levels of pain or skin problems resulting from pressure sores. Surgical contracture release procedures can facilitate hygiene, reduce pain, and improve the patient's overall quality of life.

The above mentioned situations illustrate the two main goals of orthopedic surgery. The first goal is to improve the function of the patient. The second goal is to release contractures in order to improve hygiene and to reduce pain secondary to severe spasticity. The ensuing discussion will review specific goals, candidate selection, and types of orthopedic surgery.

Functional Orthopedic Surgery

Orthopedic surgeons strive to improve the function of the patient. The function of the upper extremities includes prehension, grasp, and enabling participation in activities of daily living (ADL); the function of the spine is balanced, comfortable sitting; and the function of the lower extremities is standing and ambulation (R. R. Madigan, personal communication, November 4, 1997). Specific functional surgical goals include the following: (a) augmentation of weak muscles, (b) improvement of gross hand function, (c) improvement of grasp-release, (Roth, O'Grady, Richards, & Porte, 1993), (d) converting a nonfunctional upper extremity into an assistive extremity, (e) eliminating orthoses or enabling a patient to tolerate bracing (Jordan, 1988), (f) stabilizing joints in optimal position (R. R. Madigan, personal communication, November 4, 1997), and (g) decreasing or eliminating spasticity-induced pain.

Candidates for Functional Orthopedic Surgery

A patient is considered a candidate for orthopedic surgery to improve function if certain criteria are met in motor control, sensation, and cognitive or psychosocial categories. When evaluating motor control, the following criteria need to be considered:

1. The patient exhibits nonresponse or inadequate response to thorough trials of conservative occupational and physical therapy.

2. Gains in spontaneous neurological recovery of motor control have plateaued. This criteria specifically pertains to patients with traumatic brain injury and stroke.

3. The patient exhibits spontaneous use of the effected extremity with enough motor function to ensure a successful outcome. Dynamic polyelectromyography can be a valuable assessment tool when administered before planning orthopedic surgery (Kerrigan & Annaswamy, 1997).

4. The cause of the spastic deformities is determined as either fixed contractures or dynamic dysfunction (Braddom, 1996). To ensure surgical efficacy, static deformities must be ruled out or corrected before correcting dynamic dysfunction (Calandruccio & Jobe, 1987).

5. Other causative factors for decreased motion such as heterotopic ossification, peripheral neuropathy, disuse atrophy (Fox, 1997), fracture, fracture malunion, reflex sympathetic dystrophy, and deep vein thrombophlebitis (Hisey & Keenan, 1999) have been ruled out.

6. The state of the central nervous system (CNS) pathology is evaluated. The surgeon needs to know whether the pathology is static as in cerebral palsy or progressive as sometimes seen in multiple sclerosis (Glenn & Whyte, 1990).

The patient must have adequate sensibility to be considered an optimal candidate for functional upper extremity orthopedic surgery. The specific sensory tests include the following: (a) intact pain, temperature, and light touch; (b) 2-point discrimination less than 10 mm; and (c) kinesthetic or proprioceptive awareness (Hisey & Keenan 1999; Roper, 1987). Patients with some sensory loss can benefit from lower extremity procedures, such as the SPLATT (F. Bennett, personal communication, May 23, 1997).

Patients need to have adequate cognitive skills and a supportive network of caregivers to participate in pre- and postoperative treatment protocols. Patients need to be of a developmental age where they can cooperate and must be able to follow simple commands, remember techniques taught from one session to another, and incorporate newly learned skills into ADL (Hisey & Keenan, 1999). Furthermore, the patient has to have competent and supportive caregivers to carry out postoperative care (Glenn & Whyte, 1990).

Types of Functional Orthopedic Surgery

Soft tissue surgery. There are infinite numbers of possibilities of surgeries in the field of orthopedic spasticity management. The surgeon will often perform various combinations of releases, lengthenings, and tendon transfers in one extremity. For simplicity's sake, the authors will outline basic examples of tendon lengthening, tendon transfer, functional neurectomy, and muscle or tendon release. General postoperative therapy protocols will be referenced. The authors urge readers to discuss specific postoperative protocols with the surgeon before the initiation of therapy.

Tendon lengthening. Tendons are lengthened to diminish deforming forces by rebalancing the agonist–antagonist muscle groups or by reducing the spastic muscle's mechanical advantage (Glenn & Whyte, 1990). Tendons can be lengthened in four ways: fractional lengthening, double or triple slide cut, Z-lengthening, and V-Y technique. Surgeons gain the least amount of lengthening with fractional lengthening and the most with Z-lengthening. It is important to understand that the greater the lengthening, the greater the loss of muscle strength.

Myotendinous lengthening. Myotendinous lengthening is synonymous with fractional lengthening and muscle–tendon slide lengthening. In order to explain this technique, one must first understand the anatomy of the myotendinous junction. Some muscles have a very long insertion of the muscle into the tendon, thus there exists a portion where there is both muscle and tendon (usually the distal one third). If one cuts the tendon at the myotendinous junction, leaving the muscle intact, the whole unit will not pull apart but will gradually lengthen (R. R. Madigan, personal communication, July 31, 1997). One can typically gain up to two centimeters of lengthening using this method. Myotendinous lengthening is used whenever the anatomy of the muscle permits. This method of lengthening has several advantages. The first advantage is that fractional lengthening does not require suturing, thus minimizing the amount of scarring. The second advantage is the muscle provides a superb blood supply, which enables rapid healing.

An example of a group of muscles that can be lengthened via fractional lengthening are the wrist flexors. The tendinous portion is transected in the myotendinous junction of the flexor carpi radialis (FCR) and flexor carpi ulnaris (FCU) muscles (Figure 19). The palmaris longus muscle is released if indicated. Postoperative care involves active exercise immediately after surgery. Passive range of motion (ROM) is not permitted for 3 weeks. Resistive exercises are permitted 6 weeks after surgery (Hisey & Keenan, 1999).

Double-cut and triple-cut lengthening. The second type of tendon lengthening is known as double-cut or triple-cut lengthening. This procedure is usually performed on the Achilles tendon for the purpose of correcting an equinus deformity. For a true equinus deformity—a deformity without accompanying varus or valgus—the tendon is cut in either two or three locations. Knee and hip flexion contractures should be corrected before Achilles lengthening. The Banks and Green method of double-cut involves sectioning the anteromedial bundle distally and the posteromedial bundle proximally. All fibers are cut but at different levels. Postoperative care involves wearing a long leg cast (preferred) with the knee in extension and the ankle in neutral. Short leg casts are at times indicated, as they are more comfortable for the patient. The cast is bivalved and worn fulltime for 6 weeks to prevent the development of a calcaneus

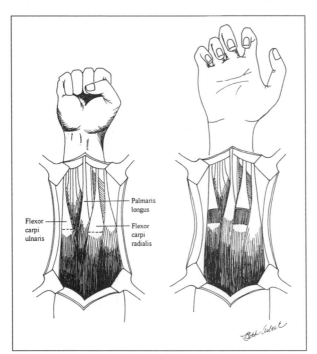

Figure 19.
Myotendinous lengthening of flexor carpi ulnaris and flexor carpi radialis. Original drawing by Beth Asbeck.

Palmaris longus

Flexor carpi ulnaris

Flexor carpi radialis

deformity. Ambulation is permitted in the cast at 1 week postsurgery. Night wear of the cast is recommended for 6 months (Glenn & Whyte, 1990).

When using the triple-cut technique, three percutaneous hemi-transections are made: the proximal incision at the musculotendinous junction, the distal hemisection near the Achilles insertion, and the center incision halfway between the proximal and distal cuts (refer to Figure 20). Postoperative care of the triple-cut method includes application of a short leg walking cast for 6 weeks. A rigid ankle foot orthoses is applied to maintain neutral foot positioning for 4 to 5 months (Keenan et al., 1993).

A complication of the Achilles lengthening procedure is over-lengthening. It can cause a calcaneous deformity in which the gait is impaired as a result of poor push off or heel to heel gait (Glenn & Whyte, 1990). The chances of this complication are decreased by following the postoperative casting and bracing protocols.

Z-lengthening. The third type of lengthening is Z-lengthening. This procedure is also known as step-cut lengthening. The surgeon gains the most length with this type of lengthening. However, the therapist and surgeon must keep in mind that the more length gained in the tendon, the weaker the muscle will become. Z-lengthening mandates suturing, thus more scarring occurs than in other procedures. Tendons have a sparse blood supply, and they heal slowly. Immobilization is required to permit the tendon to heal, therefore the onset of therapy is delayed (M. A. E. Keenan, personal communication,

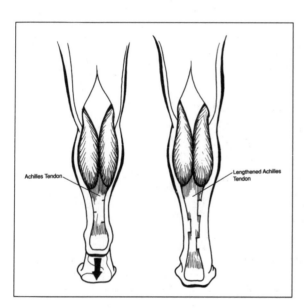

Figure 20. Triple-cut method of tendon lengthening combined with a dorsiflexion force will elongate the Achilles tendon. From M. A. E. Keenan, S. H. Kozin, & A. C. Berlet (Eds.). (1993). *Manual of orthopaedic surgery for spasticity* (p. 109). New York: Raven Press, Ltd. Reprinted with permission.

Achilles Tendon

Lengthened Achilles Tendon

August 11, 1997). Z-lengthening permits an exact amount of lengthening and is mandated if the tendon has previously undergone surgery.

Z-lengthening has been traditionally performed on the distal end of the biceps brachii tendon (Figure 21) to diminish the spastic forces of this muscle. Z-lengthening of the distal end of the biceps tendon is often performed in conjunction with a myotomy of the brachioradialis and fractional lengthening of the brachialis muscle to complete a functional elbow release procedure. Postoperative care involves casting the elbow in 45° of flexion for 4 weeks and night splint wearing for 4 more weeks. Active and passive ROM can begin after the cast is removed (Keenan et al., 1993). Recently Keenan has been lengthening the biceps from the proximal end using a myotendinous technique. This proximal lengthening technique is indicated as long as there is less than a 45° dynamic contracture at the elbow (M. A. E. Keenan, personal communication, August 11, 1997).

V-Y lengthening. The fourth type of lengthening is the V-Y technique. The V-Y technique is used to lengthen the triceps for both functional and nonfunctional neuro-orthopedic procedures. The V-Y lengthening technique can also be performed as a nonfunctional surgical procedure on the quadriceps muscle group to correct knee extension contractures (M. A. E. Keenan, personal communication, August 11, 1997). The V-Y lengthening technique is a more extensive procedure resulting in larger incisions and more extensive scarring when compared to Z-lengthening (R. R. Madigan, personal communication, July 31, 1997).

Tendon transfers. Tendon transfers serve to augment a weak or absent movement, to weaken a deforming force, or to result in a com-

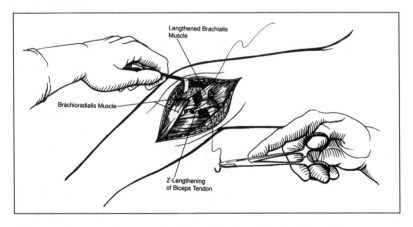

Figure 21. Z-lengthening of the biceps tendon. From M. A. E. Keenan, S. H. Kozin, & A. C. Berlet (Eds.). (1993). *Manual of orthopaedic surgery for spasticity* (p. 9). New York: Raven Press, Ltd. Reprinted with permission.

bination of both. There are several prerequisites before initiating this procedure.

1. Full preoperative passive ROM is required (Katz, 1996).

2. Usually, orthopedic surgeons prefer to transfer muscles *in-phase* whenever possible. An in-phase transfer means transferring muscles that perform a similar function, such as flexion or extension. An example of this in the hand might be transferring extensor indicis to extensor pollicis brevis. It is felt that in-phase transfers require less relearning than out-of-phase transfers. In spasticity treatment, in-phase transfers are less common as spasticity typically presents in a unilateral pulling of a limb, and all the muscles on one side may be spastic. Thus, only out-of-phase muscles may be available for transfer. Examples of a tendon transfer that could be considered in-phase commonly performed in spasticity management are the split anterior or posterior tibialis tendon transfer, profiled below (R.R. Madigan, personal communication, July 31, 1997).

3. If an in-phase transfer is not possible, an out-of-phase (also known as synergistic) transfer is advised. An example of a synergistic transfer is transferring a FCU to extensor carpi radialis longus or brevis.

4. The strength grade of the desired muscle for transfer should be good (4) or normal (5), as the muscle will usually lose one strength grade posttransfer (Calandruccio & Jobe, 1987).

5. The transferred muscle should have the same amplitude as the muscle–tendon unit it is augmenting (R. R. Madigan, personal communication, November 4, 1997).

One of the most common types of tendon transfers performed in the field of neuro-orthopedic surgery are split tendon transfers. Split tendon transfers have the advantage of augmenting the weak function without losing the primary function of the transferred tendon. An example of one of the most successful split tendon transfers is the SPLATT as shown in Figure 18. This procedure corrects a midfoot varus deformity when it is caused by spasticity in the tibialis anterior muscle (Glenn & Whyte, 1990). This procedure is often performed immediately after lengthening of the Achilles tendon and release of the toe flexors to ensure a plantigrade foot posture. The tibialis anterior tendon is split longitudinally along with a portion of its muscle belly. The lateral aspect of the tendon is attached to a hole drilled in the cuboid bone (Keenan, Kozin, & Berlet, 1993). Thus, the inversion force is reduced at the same time the eversion force is augmented, improving the balance of the foot. The SPLATT can eliminate the need for an ankle–foot orthosis (AFO), which patients often find bulky and uncomfortable to wear. Postoperative care includes the application of a short walking cast. Full weight bearing is permitted the day after surgery. The cast is worn for 6 weeks, then a rigid AFO is needed for an additional 4 to 5 months (Keenan et al., 1993).

Clinical vignette. A 24-year-old female had a spastic equinovarus deformity as a result of a stroke. She had reached maximum motor recovery. She never adjusted to her AFO, finding it uncomfortable and cosmetically unappealing. She underwent the SPLATT and lengthening of the Achilles tendon. Three months after her surgery, she did not need her AFO and was able to safely and comfortably wear sandals.

Spastic hindfoot varus is often caused from spasticity in the posterior tibialis muscle (Glenn & Whyte, 1990). Medina, Karpman, and Young (1989) split the posterior tibial tendon and attached it to the peroneus brevis tendon on 13 children with spastic cerebral palsy. Eleven children experienced excellent or good results, and two children had a fair result. Johnson and Lester (1989) studied 35 children with spastic cerebral palsy who underwent posterior tibial tendon transfer. They concluded anterior rerouting of the posterior tibial tendon was a safe and generally effective method of correcting dynamic varus deformity.

Three other noteworthy examples of functional tendon transfers are described below.

1. *Pronator to supinator transfer.* The pronator teres is detached from its insertion and transferred onto the volar aspect of the radius. This changes the pronator teres function from a forearm pronator to a forearm supinator (Roth et al., 1993).

2. *Tenodesis grasp.* Pinzur et al. (1988) studied four patients with hemiplegia who had no meaningful hand function. They developed good assistive prehensile function after undergoing a brachioradialis tendon transfer. In this procedure, the brachioradialis was detached from its insertion and attached to the extensor digitorum communis tendon. After 6 to 9 months of therapy, a tenodesis grasp was achieved (finger flexion accomplished with wrist extension and finger extension accomplished with wrist flexion).

3. *FCU transfer to extensor carpi radialis brevis or longus tendons.* The FCU tendon can be transferred to the extensor surface for

the purpose of removing a deforming force of flexion and ulnar deviation. The FCU tendon is detached from its insertion on the pisiform bone. The extensor carpi radialis brevis tendon is selected if more central wrist extension action is desired. Extensor carpi radialis longus tendon is selected if supination and wrist radial deviation is desired. The latter example accomplishes two goals. It weakens the deforming force (wrist flexion) and strengthens or augments the desired function—extension of the wrist and supination of the forearm.

4. The FCU tendon can also be transferred to the extensor digitorum communis tendon to enhance release. This is warranted when finger extension is weak, and when electromyography (EMG) reveals activity of the FCU during the release phase (Jobe, 1998).

Functional release. Releases of the muscles (myotomy) or tendons (tenotomy) are performed with a goal of eliminating a deforming force caused by severe spasticity (Katz, 1996). An example of a functional elbow release will be outlined, as this is a common deformity therapists encounter. Dynamic electromyographic studies of patients with stroke and traumatic brain injury have demonstrated that the brachioradialis exhibits severe constant spasticity, the biceps brachii has moderate spasticity, and the brachialis exhibits relatively mild spasticity (Hisey & Keenan, 1999). To gain functional elbow extension, a complete release of the brachioradialis can be performed. The brachioradialis myotomy is performed distal to the elbow, as shown in Figure 22. Along with this procedure, the biceps can be fractionally lengthened at the proximal end (M. A. E. Keenan personal communication, August 11, 1997), or Z-lengthened at the distal end, as Figure 21 demonstrates. The brachialis muscle is then lengthened via fractional lengthening (Keenan et al., 1993).

Another noteworthy functional release procedure can be performed to remedy the "thumb-in-palm" deformity. The flexor pollicis brevis and opponens pollicis are released. A Moberg screw is implanted in the interphalangeal joint to enhance lateral pinch (Keenan et al., 1993).

For other examples of functional neuro-orthopedic surgery, refer to the *Manual of Orthopedic Surgery for Spasticity* by Keenan et al. (1993). This textbook also provides examples of postoperative therapy protocols. For details focusing on upper extremity surgery, refer to Hisey and Keenan (1999), "Orthopedic management of upper extremity dysfunction following stroke or traumatic brain injury" in Green's (1999, 4th ed.) *Operative Hand Surgery*.

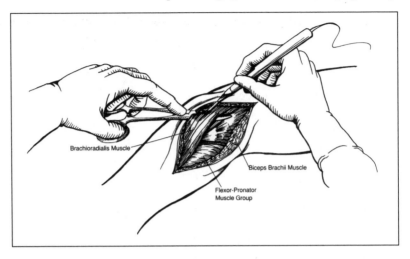

Figure 22. Myotomy of brachioradialis. From M. A. E. Keenan, S. H. Kozin, & A. C. Berlet (Eds.). (1993). *Manual of orthopaedic surgery for spasticity* (p. 7). New York: Raven Press, Ltd. Reprinted with permission.

Neurectomy. Neurectomy is defined as the surgical excision of a nerve. To manage local spasticity, the motor branches of a nerve are excised after the location is confirmed with electrical stimulation. Electrical stimulation is also used to confirm the efficacy of the neurectomy after the procedure is performed (Keenan, Todderrud, Henderson, & Botte, 1987). In other words, a neurectomy will eliminate the deforming force, as the spastic muscle will no longer have motor innervation (Braddom, 1996).

Neurectomy is a procedure usually reserved for spasticity reduction in nonfunctional patients. However, there is a noteworthy exception to this practice. In the lower extremity, hip adduction can be reduced by neurectomy of the anterior branches of the obturator nerve that innervate the adductor brevis muscle. This procedure can decrease limb scissoring and widen the lower extremity's base of support (Glenn & Whyte, 1990; Katz, 1996).

Before surgery, a diagnostic block of the obturator nerve is performed to rule out fixed contracture of the hip. The block will also serve to evaluate the patient's gait for improved ambulation. If limb scissoring is diminished and gait has improved, and the period of neurological recovery has been reached, then obturator neurectomy is indicated (Jordon, 1988; Keenan et al., 1993). Remarkably, the procedure does not last due to either nerve regrowth or reinnervation by the other nerve branches.

Functional Bone Surgery

There are three primary types of bone surgeries that are performed to correct deformities resulting from spasticity. Derotational osteotomies improve gait via physiologically correctly the angle of progression. Derotational osteotomies are most commonly performed in children with spastic cerebral palsy in the lower extremities. Spinal fusion corrects spinal deformity that prevents comfortable sitting. Joint arthrodesis (commonly referred to as fusion) fuses the bones together to result in a more stable, functional position (R.R. Madigan, personal communication, March 18, 1998).

Contracture Release: Nonfunctional Orthopedic Surgery

Specific contracture release goals are to improve hygiene, reduce pain secondary to chronic positioning, and prevent pressure sores or skin maceration (Keenan et al., 1993). Improving cosmesis may be considered as a secondary goal; however, it may not be reimbursable (Fox, 1997). When soft tissues cannot be mobilized for long periods of time as a result of severe unidirectional pulling of spasticity, contractures can develop. *Contractures* can be defined as "fixed stiffness of soft tissue, usually involving shortening or loss of elasticity of ligaments, joint capsules, and myotendinous units" (Botte et al., 1995, p. 152). Contractures are released by one or a combination of releases of fascia, muscle–tendons, and joint capsules (R. R. Madigan, personal communication, November 4, 1997).

Candidates for Contracture Release Surgery

Virtually any patient with contractures can be a candidate for contracture release surgery. The strict guidelines of motor control, sensation, and adequate cognitive abilities are not necessary for contracture release surgery. There are many settings where occupational therapists and physical therapists will encounter patients with spasticity-induced contractures, such as home health care, outpatient clinics, hospitals, and in extended care facilities. In extended care facilities quarterly resident screenings to determine the need for occupational therapy services may be mandated by state law. During these screenings, the occupational therapist and the physical therapist may discover patients with severely contracted extremities that render proper hygiene difficult if not impossible. Therapists need to evaluate the hand, wrist, elbow, axilla, perineal area, knee, and toes. Splinting is often tried and not well tolerated by these patients secondary to pain. The occupational therapist or physical therapist can recommend these patients for an orthopedic surgical consultation and be involved in the postoperative care if surgery is deemed appropriate.

The first author had a patient who developed cellulitis as a result of an infection that started in the patient's palm. This patient kept her hand in a tightly clenched fist, secondary to severe extrinsic finger flexion spasticity, which resulted in myostatic contracture of the proximal interphalangeal (PIP) and distal interphalangeal (DIP) joints. Her fourth fingernail dug into her palm causing an open wound and subsequent infection. Splinting had been tried with this patient before the infection developing, but the patient did not tolerate this secondary to pain. This situation could have been prevented had the patient had early contracture release to open up her hand.

Peripheral neuropathy can also result from chronic spasticity. For example, compression neuropathy of the ulnar nerve can be caused from spastic elbow flexors, as can carpal tunnel syndrome from spastic wrist or finger flexors. Patients with these neuropathies can benefit from orthopedic surgery (Keenan et al., 1993).

Common Upper Extremity Contracture Release Procedures

Examples of upper extremity contracture release procedures include shoulder release, elbow release, wrist flexor release, flexor digitorum sublimis to flexor digitorum profundus tendon transfer (to remedy extrinsic finger spasticity), intrinsic release with ulnar neurectomy at Guyon's canal, and wrist arthrodesis. Three procedures that exhibit examples of releases of tendon or muscle, neurectomy, and arthrodesis will be described. Postoperative protocols will be referenced.

Shoulder release. Therapists will encounter patients with severe spastic hemiplegia as a result of stroke, traumatic brain injury, or cerebral palsy who may benefit from shoulder release surgery. Shoulder adduction and internal rotation can result from fixed contracture of any of the following muscles: pectoralis major, subscapularis, latissimus dorsi, and teres major. All four muscles are typically released to correct the deformity in a nonfunctional arm with electrocautery near their insertion on the humerus. Postoperative care involves aggressive mobilization after wound healing. Gentle ROM exercises are performed to remedy residual contracture. To prevent recurrence, the shoulder is positioned in external rotation and abduction for several months with airplane splinting (Keenan et al., 1993).

Glenn and Whyte (1990) described another method to surgically repair internal rotation or adduction contracture. To be a candidate for this procedure, the patient needs to have restricted motion; less than 45° abduction and less than 15° external rotation. The subscapularis and pectoralis major tendons are released from their humeral insertion. Passive pulleys can start 24 hr postoperatively and continue for 3 months.

Complications can result after release procedures. With time, nerves and blood vessels shrink along with the joint and soft tissue contracture. Too rapid a restoration of normal length can result in nerve damage leading to pain and dysfunction or to vasospasm leading to arterial occlusion and, rarely, limb loss. Contracture releases of large joints are major procedures with the usual inherent risks of blood loss, infection, and general anesthesia (if it is used) (F. Bennett, personal communication, May 14, 1997).

Intrinsic release with ulnar neurectomy at Guyon's canal. Intrinsic spasticity is often hidden behind the existence of extrinsic flexion spasticity. After the extrinsic finger flexor spasticity is surgically corrected either by release, flexor digitorum sublimis to flexor digitorum profundus transfer, or tendon lengthening, an intrinsic positive deformity of the hand will be present, as depicted in Figure 23. Intrinsic spasticity of the hand can be relieved via neurectomy of the motor

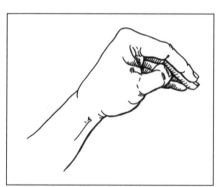

Figure 23. Intrinsic positive deformity of the hand. From M. A. E. Keenan, S. H. Kozin, & A. C. Berlet (Eds.). (1993). *Manual of orthopaedic surgery for spasticity* (p. 57). New York: Raven Press, Ltd. Reprinted with permission.

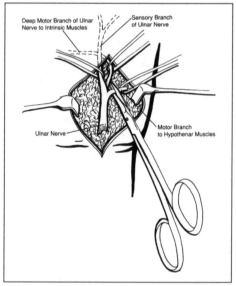

Deep Motor Branch of Ulnar Nerve to Intrinsic Muscles

Sensory Branch of Ulnar Nerve

Ulnar Nerve

Motor Branch to Hypothenar Muscles

Figure 24. Ulnar neurectomy in Guyon's canal. From M. A. E. Keenan, S. H. Kozin, & A. C. Berlet (Eds.). (1993). *Manual of orthopaedic surgery for spasticity* (p. 61). New York: Raven Press, Ltd. Reprinted with permission.

branches of the ulnar nerve in Guyon's canal, as depicted in Figure 24. This procedure accompanies the release of the intrinsic lumbrical and interossei muscles, as shown in Figure 25. The lumbrical and interossei muscles are released on both the radial and ulnar sides of the extensor mechanism on each finger and "the lateral band and oblique fibers of the extensor hood are transected on each side" (Keenan et al., 1993, p. 55).

After surgery, the hand is wrapped in a bulky dressing and immobilized for 1 week. Passive ROM can then be started. Occupational therapists should confirm with the surgeon that flexor tendon lengthening or tendon transfers have not been done concomitantly. If so, the hand and fingers are immobilized in a short arm cast for 4 weeks. Volar splinting is needed at night to prevent gravity-induced reoccurrence (Keenan et al., 1993).

Wrist arthrodesis. Joint fusion is indicated when soft tissue procedures alone are not enough to stabilize and correct deforming spastic forces (Fox, 1997; Glenn & Whyte, 1990; Katz, 1996). A type of joint fusion therapists will encounter is wrist arthrodesis. It is indicated in severe wrist flexion deformities. The goal of surgery is to permanently align the wrist in 10° to 20° of extension, which is a neutral position. The goals of arthrodesis are to relieve pain, promote stability, reduce median nerve compression, and prevent decubitus ulcers. An iliac bone graft and a 3.5 mm reconstruction plate are used to secure the fusion, as shown in Figure 26.

Postoperative management of wrist arthrodesis involves immobilizing the arm in a long splint with elevation until the edema resolves. A short arm cast is then applied for 6 to 8 weeks and is removed

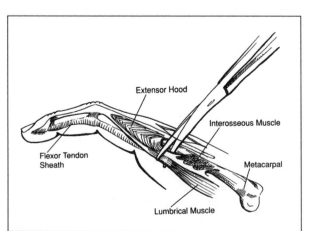

Figure 25. Release of lumbrical and interossei muscles. From M. A. E. Keenan, S. H. Kozin, & A. C. Berlet (Eds.). (1993). *Manual orthopaedic surgery for spasticity* (p. 58). New York: Raven Press, Ltd. Reprinted with permission.

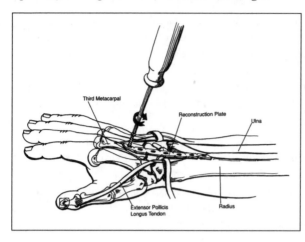

Figure 26. Wrist arthrodesis—reconstruction plate. From M. A. E. Keenan, S. H. Kozin, & A. C. Berlet (Eds.). (1993). *Manual of orthopaedic surgery for spasticity* (p. 68). New York: Raven Press, Ltd. Reprinted with permission.

when the fusion is deemed stable by X-ray examination (Keenan et al., 1993).

Hip adduction, flexion, or extension release, knee flexion or extension release, release of the plantar fascia of the foot, and triple arthrodesis of the ankle are some examples of lower extremity contracture release surgery (Katz, 1996).

Review Questions

1. Describe the difference between functional and contracture release orthopedic surgery.

2. Cerebral palsy patients who "toe-walk" may be candidates for lengthening of the _____ tendon.

3. Patient may be candidates for functional orthopedic surgery if they are still considered in a period of neurological (motor) recovery, true or false?

4. Is AROM immediately permitted after myotendinous lengthening?

5. What are the two types of functional orthopedic surgeries that can correct an equinovarus deformity?

6. To augment finger extension, what tendon can be transferred to the extensor digitorum communis tendon?

7. Which of the three elbow flexor muscles has been shown to exhibit severe spasticity upon electromyography testing?

8. Name six of the upper extremity sensory tests that therapists can perform to help aid the surgeon in candidate selection for functional orthopedic surgery.

9. Explain the difference between in-phase and out-of-phase tendon transfers. Of the two, which type is most likely performed in spasticity management?

10. Early contracture release can prevent patient suffering, decubitus ulcer development, and peripheral neuropathy, true or false?

11. What are potential complications of contracture release procedures?

12. In the nonfunctional hand, which should be corrected first—intrinsic or extrinsic spasticity?

Chapter 6

Neurosurgery in the Treatment of Spasticity: Functional Implications in Occupational and Physical Therapy

yelotomies and cordectomies are performed only on the most severe cases of spastic hypertonia and are rarely practiced. Myelotomies involve severing selected tracks of the spinal cord. Loss of bowel and bladder function may occur after myelotomy. Cordectomies involve excision of portions of the spinal cord. Cordectomies can cause severe muscle wasting and loss of bowel and bladder function (Katz, 1988).

Selective Dorsal Rhizotomy

The most common neurosurgical procedure used for spasticity is selective dorsal rhizotomy (SDR). SDR involves the cutting of dorsal spinal nerve rootlets with the primary goal of reducing spasticity in specific muscle groups. SDR is most often performed on the lumbosacral rootlets of children with spastic cerebral palsy. SDR has been performed, albeit rarely, to reduce pain and spasticity in the hemiplegic upper extremity (Katz, 1996). SDR as it pertains to pediatric cerebral palsy will be highlighted. Candidates for surgery, the surgical procedure, potential complications, and therapy postoperative protocols will be described. SDR is performed with the following goals in mind: reduce spasticity, increase range of motion (ROM), increase patient function, ease patient care, prevent the need for future orthopedic surgery (Albright, 1992), improve mobility, improve upper extremity function (Montgomery, 1992), and prevent progressive lateral migration of the femoral head of the hip (Heim, Park, Vogler, Kaufman, Noetzel, & Ortman, 1995).

Candidates

Occupational therapists and physical therapists may treat children with spastic cerebral palsy who may be candidates for SDR. Therapy evaluations are often part of the screening process that includes pediatric specialists in the following fields: neurosurgery, nursing, orthopedic surgery, physiatry, and social work (Beck, Gaskill, & Marlin, 1993). Neurosurgeons are responsible for the final decision regarding appropriate candidate selection. The following list describes factors neurosurgeons consider in determining good candidates for SDR.

1. Children 3 to 8 years of age with spastic diplegia with moderate to severe hypertonus and minimal or no ataxic or athetoid features (Katz, 1996)

2. Children who have good motor control with some degree of forward motion and whose function is believed to be limited secondary to spasticity (Katz, 1996)

3. Children with intact righting reactions (Rockman & Ploeger, 1987)

4. Children who pass computer analysis of crawling and gait (Berman, Vaughan, & Peacock, 1990)

5. Children with spasticity that hampers their ability to sit, dress, and perform perineal care (Hendricks-Ferguson & Ortman, 1995)

6. Children with an absence of significant weakness

7. Children without a significant amount of static deformity present

8. Children whose movement is not greatly influenced by the presence of primitive reflexes

9. Children with severe spasticity that causes hip dislocations and deformities that cannot be repaired with orthopedic surgery (Abbott, 1997)

In addition, patients with diplegia are better surgical candidates than those with quadriplegia (Albright, 1992; Tulipan, 1997).

The SDR selection team must also be cognizant of social, cognitive, and behavioral issues. A supportive family is needed to ensure regular therapy attendance, as well as implementation of a home postoperative positioning and exercise program (Katz, 1996). SDR is not appropriate for children who use their spasticity to walk, sit, stand, or whose functional performance would diminish without it (Albright, 1992).

Preoperative Evaluation

The authors believe standardized testing should be completed preoperatively and periodically throughout the postoperative recovery. Occupational therapists and physical therapists can be involved in the evaluation of any of the following items. Two noteworthy pediatric functional assessments include the Pediatric Evaluation of Disability Inventory[15] and the Wee Functional Independence Measure (WeeFIM®) Rating System. Therapists should consider using video tape analysis when assessing motor control (Beck, Gaskill, & Marlin, 1993; Kinghorn, 1992). The occupational therapy literature suggests that the following items should be objectively evaluated:

1. Functional fine motor skills such as reaching, grasp release, and prehension (Beck et al., 1993; Kinghorn, 1992)

2. Functional gross motor skills such as rolling, side sitting, long sitting, bench sitting, creeping, half kneeling, pulling to stand, standing, and ambulation (Beck et al., 1993; Berman, Vaughan, & Peacock, 1990)

3. Equilibrium reactions (Beck et al., 1990; Kinghorn, 1992)

4. Sensory testing

Appendix B contains the occupational therapy pediatric spasticity evaluation used before and after partial dorsal rhizotomy used at Shriners Hospital in Lexington, Kentucky. The occupational therapy evaluation is videotaped. Appendix C contains the physical therapy prerhizotomy evaluation used at Shriners Hospital in Lexington, Kentucky, and Appendix D includes the physical therapy video protocol.

Selective Dorsal Rhizotomy Procedure

SDR is usually performed on the lumbosacral rootlets. The patient is placed in a prone position and is under general anesthesia. A midline incision from L1 to S1 is made. The surgeon performs a laminotomy or laminectomy at levels L2 through L5.

The dura is opened, and the dorsal root is identified. The anterior roots are located and protected. The dorsal root is divided and rootlets are revealed (Figure 27). (Albright, 1992).The rootlets are tested with electrical stimulation. Rootlets with a normal electrical

---

[15] Pediatric Evaluation of Disability Inventory (1992). Development, standardization and administration manual, version 1.0. New England Medical Center Hospitals, Boston.

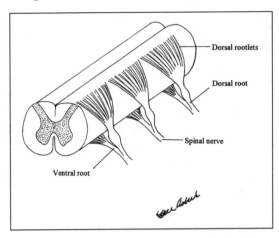

Figure 27. Spinal cord segment with rootlets. Original drawing by Beth Asbeck.

stimulation sensory threshold response are not severed. A normal response is one in which stimulation causes a local muscle to briefly contract and the effect tapers off slowly (Tulipan, 1997). Abnormal responses to stimulation are one or any of the following: (a) clonus, (b) contracture of ipsilateral muscles (i.e., muscles not typically innervated by the nerve), (c) muscle contraction that continues after the electrical stimulation has ceased (Albright, 1992), or (d) bilateral muscle contraction (Tulipan, 1997). The abnormal rootlets are severed, typically at a 10 cm distance from the spinal cord (L. Harris, personal communication, February, 1998). Typically 30% to 60% of the rootlets at levels L2 through S1 are cut. The dura is then closed, the bone excised from the laminotomy or laminectomy is replaced, and the surgical wound is closed (Albright, 1992). The onset of spasticity reduction is immediate and the duration of spasticity reduction is usually permanent, with only a 5% recurrence of spasticity (Katz, 1988).

If a partial dorsal rhizotomy is performed (as opposed to selective), the sensory rootlets are sectioned after electrical stimulation confirms that the rootlet is indeed a sensory rootlet (not a motor rootlet). An estimated 50% of the sensory rootlets are severed. Dr. Benjamin Warf, neurosurgeon at Shriners Hospital for Children, Lexington Unit, uses the above mentioned technique. For more information on his technique, refer to Warf and Nelson (1996).

Logigian, Wolinsky, Soriano, Madesen, and Scott (1994) studied 10 children with spastic cerebral palsy, 5 of whom underwent SDR, and 5 who experienced random dorsal rootlet sectioning without stimulating the sensory rootlet to determine an "abnormal" response. They concluded that spasticity reduction occurred with random partial dorsal rhizotomy, and the "current intraoperative methods for selection of abnormal dorsal rootlets may be invalid and may have no bearing on successful outcome" (Logigian et al., 1994, p. 548). This study may be limited by its small sample size.

Adverse Effects

Selective dorsal rhizotomy is a major surgical procedure, and like any other major surgery it has potential for risks. Children most commonly report "pins and needles" sensory complaints that often subside several days after surgery. Incidence of bronchospasm, aspiration pneumonia, and urinary retention has also been reported (Abbott et al., 1993; Hendricks-Ferguson, & Ortman, 1995). Bladder infection or changes in bladder control have been reported (Hendricks-Ferguson & Ortman, 1995).

There is also potential for wound infection or meningitis. Cerebrospinal fluid leakage can occur. If this happens, the child must return to surgery to locate and close the leak site. Hypotonia may also result (Albright, 1992). Infrequent potential complications involve paralysis of the legs and bladder.

Efficacy

There have been four major studies documenting changes in functional outcome after selective dorsal rhizotomy. Kinghorn (1992) followed 7 children after SDR for 1 year. Six children improved in various levels of upper-extremity function and activities of daily living (ADL), play skills, balance, and endurance. One child did not exhibit improvement in ADL. This study was limited by its small sample size. Kinghorn discussed factors that could have contributed to the observed increases in upper extremity performance. These factors included: (a) decreased spasticity as a result of the rhizotomy, (b) increased expectations of the child's family, (c) increased motivation, and (d) increased time and duration in therapy.

Berman, Vaughan, and Peacock (1990) studied 29 patients who underwent SDR for a duration of 14 months. Each patient was used as his or her own control. Significant improvements were noted in spasticity reduction, volitional movement, and joint ROM. Functional gains were noted, but they were different for each patient. The following numbers of children improved in the following areas: (a) 26 out of 29 improved in long sitting, (b) 24 out of 29 improved in half kneeling, (c) 20 out of 29 improved in their ability to roll, (d) 19 out of 29 exhibited better side sitting, and (e) 12 out of 29 improved in their ability to crawl.

Beck, Gaskill, and Marlin (1993) performed a retrospective analysis of 14 children with spastic cerebral palsy who underwent SDR. The evaluation was made before the operation and 1 year postoperatively. Statistically significant improvements were made in the assumption and maintenance of side sitting and block building.

Dudgeon and colleagues (1994) studied 29 children with spastic diplegia or quadriplegia who underwent SDR and postoperative occupational and physical therapy. The purpose of the study was to objectively evaluate improvements in specific performance skills as a result of the rhizotomy and postoperative therapy. Follow-up examinations at 6 and 12 months were completed. Patients with spastic diplegia experienced significant improvements in functional mobility and self-care. Patients with spastic quadriplegia did not make functional improvements.

A fact sheet from the United Cerebral Palsy Research and Educational Foundation (UCPREF) (1994) said of the efficacy of SDR:

> . . . there is still debate as to whether the long-term benefits of the procedure justify the risks, cost, and expenditure of family resources. At this time, the available data indicate that SDR decreases muscle tone (spasticity). However, there are inadequate data to support or reject the usefulness of selective rhizotomy to improve long-term function . . .(p. 2)

The above statement from the UCPREF still holds true today (S. Dunbar, personal communication, January 8, 1998).

Buckon, Thomas, Aiona, and Piatt (1995) supported the opinion of the UCPREF regarding lack of significant data supporting improvements in long-term function after SDR. They studied 26 children with spastic diplegia before and after selective dorsal rhizotomy to evaluate changes in upper-extremity function. No significant improvements were noted in eye–hand coordination, upper-extremity ROM, muscle tone, or strength. Grip strength did, however, increase bilaterally.

Postoperative Occupational and Physical Therapy Treatment

The following treatments are suggested in postoperative care of rhizotomy patients. This information is intended to be used as a guideline, as each patient must be progressed at their individual rate and by orders from the neurosurgeon. SDR patients usually have the following postoperative precautions:

1. Avoid passive trunk rotation for 4 weeks

2. Do not flex hips past 90°

3. Avoid hyperextension of the low back

4. Avoid sustained or excessive lumbar flexion

5. Support in sitting should be provided with 90-90-90° alignment using arm rests and foot rests. A wheelchair will be needed for at least 4 weeks postoperative (Robison, 1991).

Occupational Therapy Treatment

Occupational therapy postoperative treatment timetable may be used as a guideline. Therapists are urged to discuss postoperative protocols with the child's neurosurgeon. Appendix F includes highlights from the timetable used at Shriners Hospitals for Children, Lexington, Kentucky.

The length of hospitalization after rhizotomy varies, from 4 days to 2 weeks. Occupational and physical therapy are recommended on an outpatient basis for 1 year. Formal reevaluations are recommended at 6 months and 1 year postoperative.

Physical Therapy Postoperative Treatment

Refer to Appendix E for an example of the physical therapy postoperative assessment. Appendix G contains the physical therapy postoperative treatment protocol used at Shriners Hospital for Children, Lexington, Kentucky.

Review Questions

1. Dorsal rhizotomy is the most commonly performed neurosurgical procedure in spasticity management, true or false?

2. Name potential adverse effects that may occur after dorsal rhizotomy.

3. What is the main difference between selective and partial dorsal rhizotomy?

4. Name two standardized functional assessments that may be used by therapists pre- and postrhizotomy.

5. Name five common precautions that neurosurgeons often order after dorsal rhizotomy.

6. Name two of the four listed abnormal responses to electrical sensory rootlet stimulation.

7. It is felt dorsal rhizotomy performed on children 3 to 7 years of age may prevent the need for future orthopedic surgery, true or false?

8. Postoperative physical therapy is suggested for _____ months.

Chapter 7
Summary and Conclusions

Occupational and physical therapy professionals need to recognize when they have "met their match" in managing severe spasticity with traditional therapeutic techniques alone. Occupational therapy and physical therapy professionals can take a front-line triage role in spasticity management and make recommendations to primary care physicians to refer patients to specialists. This especially holds true when considering the effects of diagnostic-related groupings promoting earlier discharge from acute care hospitals and inpatient rehabilitation settings, as well as shortened length-of-stays due to managed care. Membership surveys conducted by the American Occupational Therapy Association (1996a, 1996b) have shown that most occupational therapy professionals now work in skilled nursing facilities and school settings where there is plenty of access to spasticity management problems and poor access to physicians skilled in spasticity treatment. These surveys also reveal that occupational therapy professionals treat stroke far more than any other diagnosis. In addition, physical therapists spend a high percentage of their time treating patients with stroke (second only to patients with low back pain).

The authors hope therapists will use the traditional therapeutic spasticity management section of this article as a quick reference. The role of physical agent modalities in spasticity was more heavily emphasized because modalities have not been comprehensively reviewed in the therapy literature with a spasticity focus. Among the various modalities, the primary author finds ultrasound helpful in inhibiting tone and aiding in patient tolerance of upper extremity functional exercise. The literature shows that functional electrical stimulation can aid in the strengthening of paretic muscles.

Occupational and physical therapists need to be familiar with oral and intrathecal antispasticity drugs, including newly released tizanidine, as well as potential side effects and adverse reactions. Phenol and botulinum toxin temporarily reduce spasticity in focal muscle groups. Phenol and botulinum toxin serve as a valuable transition between short-term and long-term spasticity management strategies, as well as have implications in easing hygiene in nonfunctional extremities. If a therapist is in doubt or fearful that a long-acting block may take away spasticity that is needed for activities of daily living participation, a short-acting block is usually a safe bet.

Selective dorsal rhizotomy has been shown to reduce tone and improve range of motion. More comprehensive occupational and physical therapy postoperative studies need to be completed to support beliefs that the patients' function has indeed improved.

Functional orthopedic surgery can be very helpful in carefully selected patients. The authors firmly believe that there is a great need for contracture release surgeries in extended care facilities.

Spasticity is a serious problem that contributes greatly to patient misery, morbidity, and dysfunction. The entire burden of every case need not rest solely on the shoulders of the treating therapist. For those patients who fail to respond to standard therapy approaches, many tools exist to help the therapist pursue better outcomes. A knowledge of available therapeutic options in the medical and surgical arenas will help the occupational and physical therapist play an even more critical role in management of the patient with spasticity, whatever its origin.

References

Abbott, R. (1997). Selective dorsal rhizotomy. *Exceptional Parent, 27*(9), 81–82.

Abbott, R., Johann-Murphy, M., Shiminski-Maher, T., Quartermain, D., Forem, S. L., Gold, J. T., & Epstein, F. J. (1993). Selective dorsal rhizotomy: Outcome and complications in treating spastic cerebral palsy. *Neurosurgery, 33*, 851–857.

Abel, N. A., & Smith, R. A. (1994). Intrathecal baclofen for treatment of intractable spinal spasticity. *Archives of Physical Medicine and Rehabilitation, 75*(1), 54–58.

Adams, R. D., & Victor, M. (1989). *Principles of neurology* (4th ed.). New York: McGraw-Hill.

Akman, M. N., Loubser, P. G., Donovan, W. H., O'Neill, M. E., & Rossi, C. D. (1993). Intrathecal baclofen: Does tolerance occur? *Paraplegia, 31*(8), 516–520.

Albright, A. L. (1992). Neurosurgical treatment of spasticity: Selective posterior rhizotomy and intrathecal baclofen. *Stereotactic and Functional Neurosurgery, 58*(1–4), 3–13.

Albright, A. L., Cervi, A., & Singletary, J. (1991). Intrathecal baclofen for spasticity in cerebral palsy. *Journal of the American Medical Association, 265*, 1418–1422.

American Occupational Therapy Association. (1996a). *Member Data Survey. Percentage of registered occupational therapists & certified occupational therapy assistants by most frequently treated health problem.* Bethesda, MD: Author.

American Occupational Therapy Association. (1996b). *Member data survey. Percentage of registered occupational therapists & certified occupational therapy assistants by primary employment setting.* Bethesda, MD: Author.

American Physical Therapy Association, Research Services. (1996). *Practice profile survey: Percentage of time spent with patients with conditions in the following areas.* Alexandria, VA: Author.

Ashworth, B. (1964). Preliminary trial of carisporodol in multiple sclerosis. *Practitioner, 192*, 540–542.

Basmajian, J. V., & DeLuca, C. J. (1985). *Muscles alive: Their functions revealed by electromyography* (5th ed.). Baltimore: Williams & Wilkins.

Beck, A. J., Gaskill, S. J., & Marlin, A. E. (1993). Improvement in upper extremity function and trunk control after selective posterior rhizotomy. *American Journal of Occupational Therapy, 47,* 704–707.

Becker, W. J., Harris, C. J., Long, M. L., Ablett, D. P., Klein, G. M., & DeForge, D. A. (1995). Long-term intrathecal baclofen therapy in patients with intractable spasticity. *Canadian Journal of Neurological Sciences, 22*(3), 208–217.

Berman, B., Vaughan, C. L., & Peacock, W. J. (1990). The effect of rhizotomy on movement in patients with cerebral palsy. *American Journal of Occupational Therapy, 44,* 511–516.

Bhakta, B. B., Cozens, J. A., Bamford, J. M., & Chamberlain, M. A. (1996). Use of botulinum toxin in stroke patients with severe upper limb spasticity. *Journal of Neurology, Neurosurgery and Psychiatry, 61*(1), 30–35.

Blumenkopf, B. (1997, May). Intrathecal baclofen for spasticity. In P. D. Charles (Chair), *Treatment advances in spasticity.* Symposium conducted at Vanderbilt University Medical Center, Nashville, TN.

Bobath, B. (1978). *Adult hemiplegia: Evaluation and treatment* (2nd ed.). London: Heinemann/Medical.

Bohannon, R. W. (1993). Tilt table standing for reducing spasticity after spinal cord injury. *Archives of Physical Medicine and Rehabilitation, 74,* 1121–1122.

Bohannon, R. W., & Smith, M. B. (1987). Interrater reliability of a modified Ashworth scale of muscle spasticity. *Physical Therapy, 67*(2), 206–207.

Bonzani, P. (1997, June). *Physical agent modalities for upper limb rehabilitation.* Paper presented at Physiotherapy Associates, Charlotte, NC.

Booth, B. J., Doyle, M., & Montgomery J. (1983). Serial casting for the management of spasticity in the head injured adult. *Physical Therapy, 63,* 1960–1966.

Borg-Stein, J., Pine, Z. M., Miller, J. R., & Brin, M. F. (1993). Botulinum toxin for the treatment of spasticity in multiple sclerosis. *American Journal of Physical Medicine and Rehabilitation, 72,* 364–368.

Botte, M. J., Abrams, R. A., & Bodine-Fowler, S. C. (1995). Treatment of acquired muscle spasticity using phenol peripheral nerve blocks. *Orthopedics, 18*(2), 151–159.

Botte, M. J., & Keenan, M. A. E. (1988). Percutaneous phenol blocks of the pectoralis major muscle to treat spastic deformities. *Journal of Hand Surgery, American Volume, 13*(1), 147–149.

Botulinum toxin approved by Medicare. *Medicare Bulletin*—GR 96-5, Tennessee insert, p. 49.

Braddom, R. L. (Ed.). (1996). *Physical medicine and rehabilitation.* Philadelphia: W. B. Saunders.

Brunnstrom, S. (1970). *Movement therapy in hemiplegia* (1st ed.). New York: Harper & Row.

Buckon, C. E., Thomas, S. S., Aiona, M. D., & Piatt, J. H. (1995). Assessment of upper-extremity function in children with spastic diplegia before and after selective dorsal rhizotomy. *Developmental Medicine and Child Neurology, 38*(11), 967–975.

Caine, S. (1993). Local treatment of dystonia and spasticity with injections of botulinum-A toxin. *AXONE, 14*(4), 85–88.

Calandruccio, J. H., & Jobe, M. T. (1987). Paralytic hand. In A. H. Crenshaw (Ed.), *Campbell's operative orthopaedics* (8th ed., pp. 3233–3243). St. Louis: Mosby-Year Book, Inc.

Carmick, J. (1993). Clinical use of neuromuscular electrical stimulation for children with cerebral palsy, part 2: Upper extremity. *Physical Therapy, 73*(8), 514–527.

Carmick, J. (1995). Managing equinus in children with cerebral palsy: Electrical stimulation to strengthen the triceps surae muscle. *Developmental Medicine and Child Neurology, 37*(11), 965–975.

Chakerian, D. L., & Larson, M. A. (1993). Effects of upper-extremity weight-bearing on hand-opening and prehension patterns in children with cerebral palsy. *Developmental Medicine and Child Neurology, 35*(3), 216–229.

Charles, P. D. (1997, May). Botox for spasticity. In P. D. Charles (Chair), *Treatment advances in spasticity.* Symposium conducted at Vanderbilt University Medical Center, Nashville, TN.

Cherry, D. B., & Weigand, G. M. (1981). Plaster drop-out casts as a dynamic means to reduce muscle contracture. *Physical Therapy, 61*(11), 1601–1603.

Chironna, R. L., & Hecht, J. S. (1990). Subscapularis motor point block for the painful hemiplegic shoulder. *Archives of Physical Medicine and Rehabilitation, 71*(6), 428–429.

References

Cruickshank, D. A., & O'Neill, D. L. (1990). Upper-extremity inhibitive casting in a boy with spastic quadriplegia. *American Journal of Occupational Therapy, 44,* 552–555.

Currie, D. M., & Mendiola, A. (1987). Cortical thumb orthosis for children with spastic hemiplegic cerebral palsy. *Archives of Physical Medicine and Rehabilitation, 68*(4), 214–216.

Das, T. K., & Park, D. M. (1989). Botulinum toxin in treating spasticity. *British Journal of Clinical Practice, 43*(11), 401–403.

Davis, J. Z. (1996). Neurodevelopmental treatment of adult hemiplegia: The Bobath approach. In L. W. Pedretti (Ed.), *Occupational therapy practice skills for physical dysfunction* (4th ed., pp. 435–450). St Louis: Mosby-Year Book.

Dee, R. (1969). Structure and function of hip joint innervation. *Annals of the Royal College of Surgeons of England, 45,* 357–374.

Doraisamy, P. (1992). The management of spasticity—A review of options available in rehabilitation. *Annals Academy of Medicine, Singapore, 21,*(6) 807–812.

Dudgeon, M. S., Libby, A. K., McLaughlin, J. F., Hays, R. M., Bjornson, M. S., & Roberts, T. S. (1994). Prospective measurement of functional changes after selective dorsal rhizotomy. *Archives of Physical Medicine and Rehabilitation, 75*(1), 46–53.

Eltorai, I., & Montroy, R. (1990). Muscle release in the management of spasticity in spinal cord injury. *Paraplegia, 28*(7), 433–440.

Feldman, P. A. (1990). Upper extremity casting and splinting. In M. B. Glenn, & J. Whyte (Eds.). *The Practical management of spasticity in children and adults* (pp. 149–200). Philadelphia: Lea & Febiger.

Fox, J. (1997, May). Orthopedic options. In P. D. Charles (chair), *Treatment advances in spasticity.* Symposium conducted at Vanderbilt University Medical Center, Nashville, TN.

Gardner, B., Jamous, A., Teddy, P., Bergstrom, E., Wang, D., Ravichandran, G., Sutton, R., & Urquart, S. (1995). Intrathecal baclofen—A multicentre clinical comparison of the Medtronics Programmable, Cordis Secor, and Constant Infusion Infusaid drug delivery systems. *Paraplegia, 33,* 551–554.

Garland, D. E., Lilling, M., & Keenan, M. A. E. (1984). Percutaneous phenol blocks to motor points of spastic forearm muscles in head-injured adults. *Archives of Physical Medicine and Rehabilitation, 65,* 243–245.

Geiringer, S. R. (1994). *Anatomic location for needle electromyography.* Philadelphia: Hanley & Belfus.

Gerszten, P. C., Albright, A. L., & Johstone, G. F. (1998). Intrathecal baclofen infusion and subsequent orthopedic surgery in patients with spastic cerebral palsy. *Journal of Neurosurgery, 88,* 1009–1013.

Gianino, J. (1993). Intrathecal baclofen for spinal spasticity: Implications for nursing practice. *Journal of Neuroscience Nursing, 25(4),* 254–264.

Giebler, K. B. (1990). Physical modalities. In M. B. Glenn & J. Whyte (Eds.). *The practical management of spasticity in children and adults* (pp. 118–148). Philadelphia: Lea & Febiger.

Glenn, M. B. (1990). Nerve blocks. In M. B. Glenn & J. Whyte (Eds.). *The practical management of spasticity in children and adults* (pp. 227–258). Philadelphia: Lea & Febiger.

Glenn, M. B., & Elovic, E. (1997). Chemical denervation for the treatment of hypertonia and related motor disorders: Phenol and botulinum toxin. *Journal of Head Trauma Rehabilitation, 12(6),* 40–62.

Glenn, M. B., & Whyte, J. (Eds.). (1990). *The practical management of spasticity in children and adults.* Philadelphia: Lea & Febiger.

Goff, B. (1976). Grading of spasticity and its effect on voluntary movement. *Physiotherapy, 62,(11),* 358–361.

Gooch, J. L., & Sandell, T. V. (1996). Botulinum toxin for spasticity and athetosis in children with cerebral palsy. *Archives of Physical Medicine and Rehabilitation, 77(5),* 508–511.

Goodman, G., & Bazyk, S. (1991). The effects of a short thumb opponens splint on hand function in cerebral palsy: A single subject study. *American Journal of Occupational Therapy, 45,* 726–731.

Grazko, M. A., Polo, K. B., & Jabbari, B. (1995). Botulinum toxin A for spasticity, muscle spasms, and rigidity. *Neurology, 45(4),* 712–717.

Green, D. P., Hotchkiss, R., & Pederson, W. C. (1999). *Green's operative hand surgery* (4th ed.). New York: Churchill Livingstone.

Greenbaum, M. G., Young, M. A., & Frank, J. M. (1993). Attenuation of facial muscle spasticity with intramuscular phenol neurolysis. *Archives of Physical Medicine and Rehabilitation, 74(2),* 217–219.

Hardman, J. G., & Limbird, L. E. (Eds.). (1995). *Goodman and Gilman's the pharmacological basis of therapeutics* (9th ed.). New York: McGraw-Hill.

Hecht, J. S. (1992). Subscapular nerve block in the painful hemiplegic shoulder. *Archives of Physical Medicine and Rehabilitation, 73(11),* 1036–1039.

Heim, R. C., Park, T. S., Vogler, G. P., Kaufman, B. A., Noetzel, M. J., & Ortman, M. R. (1995). Changes in hip migration after selective dorsal rhizotomy for spastic quadriplegia in cerebral palsy. *Journal of Neurosurgery, 82*(4), 567–571.

Hendricks-Ferguson, V. L., & Ortman, M. R. (1995). Selective dorsal rhizotomy to decrease spasticity in cerebral palsy. *AORN Journal, 61*(3), 514–518, 521–522, 525.

Hesse, S., Lücke, D., Malezic, M., Bertelt, C., Friedrich, H., Gregoric, M., & Mauritz, K. H. (1994). Botulinum toxin treatment for lower limb extensor spasticity in chronic hemiparetic patients. *Journal of Neurology, Neurosurgery, and Psychiatry, 57*(11), 1321–1324.

Hill, J. (1994). The effects of casting on upper-extremity motor disorders after brain injury. *American Journal of Occupational Therapy, 48,* 219–224.

Hinderer, S. R., & Gupta, S. (1996). Methods and scales of functional outcome measures to assess interventions for spasticity. *Archives of Physical Medicine and Rehabilitation, 77,* 1083–1088.

Hines, A. E., Crago, P. E., & Billian, C. (1993). Functional electrical stimulation for the reduction of spasticity in the hemiplegic hand. *Biomedical Sciences Instrumentation, 29,* 259–266.

Hisey, M. S., & Keenan, M. A. E. (1999). Orthopaedic management of upper extremity dysfunction following stroke or brain injury. In D. P. Green, R. Hotchkiss, & W.C. Pederson (Eds.), *Operative hand surgery* (4th ed., pp. 287–324). New York: Churchill Livingstone.

Hylton, N. (1990). Dynamic casting and orthotics. In M. B. Glenn & J. Whyte (Eds.). *The practical management of spasticity in children and adults* (pp. 167–200). Philadelphia: Lea & Febiger.

Intiso, D., Santilli, V., Grasso, M. G., Rossi, R., & Caruso, I. (1994). Rehabilitation of walking with electromyographic biofeedback in foot-drop after stroke. *Stroke, 25,* 1189–1192.

Jobe, M. T. (1998). Cerebral palsied hand. In S. T. Canale (Ed.) *Campbell's operative orthopedics* (9th ed., pp. 3593–3604). St. Louis: Mosby.

Joe, B, E. (1996, October 31). Hand mobility restored 20 years after accident. *OT Week,* 16–17.

Johnson, J., & Vernon, D. (1992, June). Elastic tubular bandages: An adjunctive treatment approach to abnormal muscle tone. *Gerontology Special Interest Section Newsletter, 15*(2), 3–4.

Johnson, W. L., & Lester, E. L. (1989). Transposition of the posterior tibial tendon. *Clinical Orthopaedics and Related Research, 245,* 223–227.

Jordan, C. (1988). Current status of functional lower extremity surgery in adult spastic patients. *Clinical Orthopaedics and Related Research, 233,* 102–109.

Katz, R. T. (1988). Management of spasticity. *American Journal of Physical Medicine and Rehabilitation, 67*(3), 108–116.

Katz, R. T. (1996). Management of spasticity. In R. L. Braddom (Ed.). *Physical medicine and rehabilitation* (1st ed., pp. 580–604). Philadelphia: W. B. Saunders.

Keenan, M. A. E. (1987). The orthopedic management of spasticity. *Journal of Head Trauma Rehabilitation, 2*(2), 62–71.

Keenan, M. A. E., Korchek, J. I., Botte, M. J., Smith, C. W., & Garland, D. E. (1987). Results of transfer of the flexor digitorum superficialis tendons to the flexor digitorum profundus tendons in adults with acquired spasticity of the hand. *Journal of Bone and Joint Surgery, American Volume, 69,* 1127–1132.

Keenan, M. A. E., Kozin, S. H., & Berlet, A. C. (1993). *Manual of orthopedic surgery for spasticity.* New York: Raven Press.

Keenan, M. A. E., Todderud, E. P., Henderson, R., & Botte, M. (1987). Management of intrinsic spasticity in the hand with phenol injection or neurectomy of the motor branch of the ulnar nerve. Part 1. *Journal of Hand Surgery, American Volume, 12*(5), 734–739.

Keenan, M. A. E., Tomas, E. S., Stone, L., & Gersten, L. M. (1990). Percutaneous phenol block of the musculocutaneous nerve to control elbow flexor spasticity. *Journal of Hand Surgery, American Volume, 15*(2), 340–346.

Kerrigan, D. C., & Annaswamy, T. M (1997). The functional significance of spasticity as assessed by gait analysis. *Journal of Head Trauma Rehabilitation, 12*(6), 29–39.

King, T. I., II (1982). Plaster splinting as a means of reducing elbow flexor spasticity. *American Journal of Occupational Therapy, 36,* 671–673.

King, T. I., II (1996). The effect of neuromuscular electrical stimulation in reducing tone. *American Journal of Occupational Therapy, 50,* 62–64.

Kinghorn, J. (1992). Upper extremity functional changes following selective posterior rhizotomy in children with cerebral palsy. *American Journal of Occupational Therapy, 46,* 502–507.

Kisner, C., & Colby, L. A. (1996). *Therapeutic exercise foundations and techniques.*(3rd ed., pp. 149–150). Philadelphia: F. A. Davis.

Knott, M., & Voss, D. E. (1956). *Proprioceptive neuromuscular facilitaion: Patterns and techniques.* New York: Hoeber Medical Division, Harper & Row.

Koman, L. A., Mooney, J. F., III, Smith, B., Goodman, A., & Mulvaney, T. (1993). Management of cerebral palsy with botulinum-A toxin: Preliminary investigation. *Journal of Pediatric Orthopedics, 13*(4), 489–495.

Koman, L. A., Mooney, J. F., III, Smith, B. P., Goodman, A., & Mulvaney, T. (1994). Management of spasticity in cerebral palsy with botulinum-A toxin: Report of a preliminary, randomized, double-blind trial. *Journal of Pediatric Orthopedics, 14*(3), 299–303.

Langlois, S., MacKinnon, J. R., & Pederson, L. (1989). Hand splints and cerebral spasticity: A review of the literature. *Canadian Journal of Occupational Therapy, 56*(3), 113–119.

Langlois, S., Pederson, L., & MacKinnon, J. R. (1991). The effects of splinting on the spastic hemiplegic hand: Report of a feasibility study. *Canadian Journal of Occupational Therapy, 58*(1), 17–25.

Lazorthes, Y., Sallerin-Caute, B., Verdie, J. C., Bastide, R., & Carillo, J. P. (1990). Chronic intrathecal baclofen administration for control of severe spasticity. *Journal of Neurosurgery, 72*(3), 393–402.

Little, J. W., & Massagli, T. L. (1998). Spasticity and associated abnormalities of muscle tone. In J. A. DeLisa & B. M. Gans (Eds.), *Rehabilitation medicine: Principles and practice* (3rd ed., pp. 997–999). Philadelphia: Lippincott-Raven.

Logigian, E. L., Wolinsky, J. S., Soriano, S. G., Madsen, J. R., & Scott, R. M. (1994). H reflex studies in cerebral palsy patients undergoing partial dorsal rhizotomy. *Muscle and Nerve, 17*(5), 539–549.

McCormack, G. L. (1996). The Rood approach to treatment of neuromuscular dysfunction. In L. W. Pedretti (Ed.). *Occupational therapy practice skills for physical dysfunction* (4th ed., pp. 377–399). St. Louis: Mosby–Year Book, Inc..

McCormack, G. L., & Feuchter, F. (1996). Neurophysiology for the sensorimotor approaches to treatment. In L. W. Pedretti (Ed.), *Occupational therapy practice skills for physical dysfunction* (4th ed., p. 366). St. Louis: Mosby–Year Book, Inc.

McCormack, G. L., & Pedretti, L. W. (1996). Motor unit dysfunction. In L. W. Pedretti (Ed.), *Occupational therapy practice skills for physical dysfunction* (4th ed., pp. 747–761). St. Louis: Mosby–Year Book, Inc.

McPherson, J. J. (1981). Objective evaluation of a splint designed to reduce hypertonicity. *American Journal of Occupational Therapy, 35*, 189–194.

McPherson, J. J., Kreimeyer, D., Aalderks, M., & Gallagher, T. (1982). A comparison of dorsal and volar resting hand splints in the reduction of hypertonus. *American Journal of Occupational Therapy, 36*, 664–670.

Medina, P. A., Karpman, R. R., & Yeung, A. T. (1989). Split posterior tibial tendon transfer for spastic equinovarus foot deformity. *Foot and Ankle, 10*(2), 65–67.

Milazzo, S. & Gillen, G. (1998). Splinting applications. In Gillen & Burkhardt (Eds.), *Stroke rehabilitation: A function-based approach* (pp. 161–184). St. Louis: Mosby–Year Book, Inc.

Montgomery, P. C. (1992). A clinical report of long-term outcomes following selective posterior rhizotomy: Implications for selection, follow-up and research. *Physical and Occupational Therapy in Pediatrics, 12*(1), 69–87.

Moore, T. J., & Anderson, R. B. (1991). The use of open phenol blocks to the motor branches of the tibial nerve in adult acquired spasticity. *Foot and Ankle, 11*(4), 219–221.

Morrison, J. E., Jr., Matthews, D., Washington, R., Fennessey, P. V., & Harrison, L. M. (1991). Phenol motor point blocks in children: Plasma concentrations and cardiac dysrhythmias. *Anesthesiology, 75*(2), 359–362.

National Spinal Cord Statistical Center. (1998). *Spinal cord injury facts and figures at a glance, January, 1998*. Birmingham, AL: Author.

Ottenbacher, K. (1983). Developmental implications of clinically applied vestibular stimulation. *Physical Therapy, 63*, 338–342.

Ottenbacher, K., Short, M. A., & Watson, P. J. (1981). The effects of a clinically applied program of vestibular stimulation on the neuromotor performance of children with severe developmental disability. *Physical and Occupational Therapy in Pediatrics, 1*(3), 1–11.

Pape, K. E. (1994). Caution urged for NMES use [Letter to the editor]. *Physical Therapy, 74*(3), 265–267.

Patricia Neal Rehabilitation Center Policy and Procedure Manual (1998). [Available from 1901 Clinch Avenue, Knoxville, TN 37916].

Pedretti, L. W. (1985). *Occupational therapy practice skills for physical dysfunction* (2nd ed.). St. Louis: Mosby-Year Book, Inc.

Pedretti, L. W. (1996). *Occupational therapy practice skills for physical dysfunction* (4th ed.). St. Louis: Mosby-Year Book, Inc.

Petrillo, C. R., & Knoploch, S. (1988). Phenol block of the tibial nerve for spasticity: A long-term follow-up study. *International Disability Studies, 10*(3), 97–100.

Physicians desk reference (52nd ed.). (1998). Montvale, NJ: Medical Economics Company.

Pierson, S. H., Katz, D. I., & Tarsy, D. (1996). Botulinum toxin A in the treatment of spasticity: Functional implications and patient selection. *Archives of Physical Medicine and Rehabilitation, 77*(7), 717–721.

Pinzur, M. S., Wehner, J., Kett, N., & Trilla, M.(1988). Brachioradialis to finger extensor tendon transfer to achieve hand opening in acquired spasticity. *Journal of Hand Surgery, American Volume, 13*, 549–552.

Rawlins, P. (1995). Intrathecal baclofen for spasticity of cerebral palsy: Project coordination and nursing care. *Journal of Neuroscience Nursing, 27*(3), 157–163.

Robison, J. (1997, May). Physical therapy for spasticity. In P. D. Charles (Chair). *Treatment advances in spasticity*. Symposium conducted at Vanderbilt University Medical Center, Nashville, TN.

Rockman, R. C., & Ploeger, D. N. (1987, September). Consideration for selective posterior rhizotomy. *Developmental Disabilities Special Interest Section Newsletter, 10*(3), 8.

Rood, M. (1962). The use of sensory receptors to activate, facilitate, and inhibit motor response, autonomic and somatic, in developmental sequence. In C. Sattely (Ed.), *Approaches to the treatment of patients with neuromuscular dysfunction*. Dubuque, IA: Wm. C. Brown Book.

Roper, B. A. (1987). The orthopedic management of the stroke patient. *Clinical Orthopaedics and Related Research, 219*, 78–85.

Rose, V., & Shah, S. (1987). A comparative study on the immediate effects of hand orthoses on reduction of hypertonus. *Australian Occupational Therapy Journal, 34*(2), 59–64.

Roth, J. H., O'Grady, S. E., Richards, R. S., & Porte, A. M. (1993). Functional outcome of upper limb tendon transfers performed in children with spastic hemiplegia. *Journal of Hand Surgery, British Volume, 18*(3), 299–303.

Savoy, S. M., & Gianino, J. M. (1993). Intrathecal baclofen infusion: An innovative approach for controlling spinal spasticity. *Rehabilitation Nursing, 18*(2), 105–113.

Siegfried, R. N., Jacobson, L., & Chabal, C. (1992). Development of an acute withdrawal syndrome following the cessation of intrathecal baclofen in a patient with spasticity. *Anesthesiology, 77*(5), 1048–1050.

Simpson, D. M., Alexander, D. N., O'Brien, C. F., Tagliati, M., Aswad, A. S., Leon, J. M., Gibson, J., Mordaunt, J. M., & Monaghan, E. P. (1996). Botulinum toxin type A in the treatment of upper extremity spasticity: A randomized, double-blind, placebo-controlled trial. *Neurology, 46*, 1306–1310.

Snook, J. H. (1979). Spasticity reduction splint. *American Journal of Occupational Therapy, 33*, 648–651.

Snow, B. J., Tsui, J. K., Bhatt, M. H., Varelas, M., Hashimoto, S. A., & Calne, D. B. (1990). Treatment of spasticity with botulinum toxin: A double-blind study. *Annals of Neurology, 28*(4), 512–515.

Swaan, D., van Wieringen, P. C., & Fokkema, S. D. (1974). Auditory electromyographic feedback therapy to inhibit undesired motor activity. *Archives of Physical Medicine and Rehabilitation, 55*(6), 251–254.

Trombly, C. A. (Ed.). (1983). *Occupational therapy for physical dysfunction* (2nd ed.). Baltimore: Williams & Wilkins.

Trombly, C. A., & Scott, A. D. (1977). *Occupational therapy for physical dysfunction*, Baltimore: Williams & Wilkins.

Tulipan, N. (1997, May). Neurosurgical options. In P. D. Charles (Chair), *Treatment advances in spasticity*. Symposium conducted at Vanderbilt University Medical Center, Nashville, TN.

Twist, D. J. (1985). Effects of a wrapping technique on passive ROM in a spastic upper extremity. *Physical Therapy, 65*, 299–304.

Umphred, D. A. (Ed.), (1995). *Neurological rehabilitation* (3rd ed.). St. Louis: Mosby–Year Book.

United Cerebral Palsy Research and Educational Foundation. (1994, February). *Selective dorsal rhizotomy a neurosurgical approach to muscle spasticity* [Research fact sheet], 1–2.

Wassef, M. R. (1993). Interadductor approach to obturator nerve blockade for spastic conditions of adductor thigh muscles. *Regional Anesthesia, 18*(1), 13–17.

Werner, J. K. (1980). *Neuroscience, a clinical perspective*. Philadelphia: W. B. Saunders.

Wilson, D. S. (1997, June). Spasticity: Its management with neuroablative phenolization. *Gerontology Special Interest Section Newsletter, 15*(2), 1–3.

Yablon, S. A., Agana, B. T., Ivanhoe, C. B., & Boake, C. (1996). Botulinum toxin in severe upper extremity spasticity among patients with traumatic brain injury: An open-labeled trial. *Neurology, 47,* 939–944.

Yadav, S. L., Singh, U., Dureja, G. P., Singh, K. K., & Chaturvedi, S. (1994). Phenol block in the management of cerebral palsy. *Indian Journal of Pediatrics, 61*(3), 249–255.

Yasukawa, A. (1990). Upper-extremity casting: Adjunct treatment for a child with cerebral palsy hemiplegia. *American Journal of Occupational Therapy, 44,* 840–846.

Young, R. R. (1994). Spasticity: A review. *Neurology, 44*(Suppl. 9), S12–S20.

Resources

1. ADL & Rehabilitation catalog, North Coast Medical, 18305 Sutter Boulevard, Morgan Hill, CA 95037-2845; 800-821-9319; www.ncmedical.com

2. Contractures: Orthotic Management of Contracture and Spasticity, AliMed®, 297 High Street, Dedham, MA 02026; 800-225-2610; www.alimed.com

3. EMPI, P.O. Box 709, Clear Lake, SD 57226; 800-328-2536; www.EMPI.com

4. Product Catalog, DeRoyal/LMB, 200 DeBusk Lane, Powell, TN 37849; 800-541-3992; www.dewab.com

5. Rehabilitation Division, Smith & Nephew, Inc., One Quality Drive, P.O. Box 1005, Germantown, WI 53022-8205; 800-558-8633; www.easyliving.com

6. R S Medical, 14401 S.E. First Street, Vancouver, WA 98684-3503; 360-892-0339

7. Sammons™–Preston, P.O. Box 5071, Bolingbrook, IL 60440-5071; 800-323-5547; www.sammonspreston.com

Appendix A
Patricia Neal Rehabilitation Center
Occupational/Physical Therapy Spasticity Evaluation

Patient Name: _____

Patient #: _____

1. SUBJECTIVE

A. Patient's or family's chief concerns regarding spasticity: _____

_____

B. Does spasticity interfere with function, positioning, or caregiving? _____

_____

C. Pain rating scale (Key: 0 = no pain, 10 = severe enough to warrant hospitalization) _____

D. History of previous therapy, medical, or surgical spasticity treatment _____

_____

E. Medications _____

2. OBJECTIVE

A. Sensation: Static 2-point discrimination _____

Semmes-Weinstein monofilaments[1] _____

5 item stereognosis _____

Kinesthesia/Proprioception _____

Comments _____

B. Spasm frequency score (Snow et al., 1990) _____

Key: 0 = no spasms

1 = one or fewer spasms per day

2 = between 1 and 5 spasms per day

3 = between 5 to 9 spasms per day

4 = 10 or more spasms per day, or continuous contraction

C. Grip/pinch:

	R or L	Norms
Grip strength	_____	_____
Palmar pinch	_____	_____
Lateral pinch	_____	_____
Tip pinch	_____	_____

---

[1] North Coast™ Medical, Inc., 187 Stauffer Blvd., San Jose, CA 95125

D. Upper Extremity Range of Motion Evaluation

Right _____   Left _____

MOTION TESTED		AROM	PROM
UPPER EXTREMITY	NORMS IN DEGREES		
SHOULDER			
Shld Ext/Flex	60/180		
Shld Abd/Add	180/0		
Shld Hor. Abd/Add	90/45		
Shld IR/ER	70/90		
Scaption	0–180°		
ELBOW/FOREARM and WRIST			
Elbow Ext/Flex	0/150		
Forearm Sup/Pron.	80/80		
Wrist Ext/Flex	30/20		
Ulnar/Radial Dev.	30/20		
THUMB			
CMC Flex	0/50		
CMC Retroposition	7 cm		
MP Ext/Flex	+20/60		
IP Ext/Flex	+30/80		
Opposition	8 cm		
Addiction	2 cm		
Radical Abduction	0/50		
Palmar Abduction	0/50		
SECOND DIGIT			
MP Ext/Flex	+20/90		
PIP	0/100		
DIP	0/70		

MOTION TESTED		AROM	PROM
THIRD DIGIT	NORMS IN DEGREES		
MP Ext-Flex	+20/90		
PIP	0/100		
DIP	0/70		
FOURTH DIGIT			
MP Ext/Flex	+20/90		
PIP	0/100		
DIP	0/70		
FIFTH DIGIT			
MP Ext/Flex	+20/90		
PIP	0/100		
DIP	0/70		
LOWER EXTREMITY			
HIP			
Ext/Flex	30/120		
Abduction	0/45		
Adduction	0/30		
IR/ER	45/45		
KNEE			
Ext/Flex	0/135		
ANKLE			
Dorsiflexion	0/20		
Plantarflexion	0/50		
Inversion	0/35		
Eversion	0/15		

E. Gait evaluation (general description) _____

_____

Device _____   Deviation _____
Sit to stand _____   Swing phase _____
Stance phase_____   Synergy patterns _____
Distance _____   Speed _____

F. Balance _____
Sitting _____
Standing _____

G. FIM™ instrument scoring for levels of assistance[2]

No Helper

    7 = complete independence

    6 = modified independence (equipment)

Helper

    5 = supervison (set up, cueing or learning)

    4 = minimal assistance

    3 = moderate assistance

    2 = maximal assistance

    1 = total assistance

_____

_____

_____

_____

H. Narrative description of muscle tone (synergy present/primitive reflexes present?) _____

_____

_____

_____

3. QUANTIFICATION OF MUSCLE TONE AND STRENGTH

Muscle Tone Key:

Flaccid = no tone, no active movement

Paretic = weak, some active movement

*Trombly & Scott (1977) Spasticity Scale

**Mild* = if the stretch reflex occurs when the muscle is in a lengthened position,

**Moderate* = if it occurs in the middle of the range,

* *Severe* = if it occurs when the muscle is in a shortened range.

Clonus = repetitive rhythmic contractions/relaxations

Rigidity = increased resistance to passive stretch throughout the range of motion (both agonist and antagonist)

Strength key: 0 = no m. contraction

            1 = m. contraction palpated, no joint movement

            2 = full ROM, gravity-reduced plane

            3 = full ROM, against gravity

            4 = moderate resistance tolerated

            5 = normal strength

Muscle or Muscle group	Tone in supine	Tone in sitting	Tone in standing or walking	Muscle strength grade[3]
SCAPULA				
Elevators				
Depressors				
Retractors				
Protractors				
Scaption				
SHOULDER				
Flexors				
Extensors				
Adductors				
Abductors				
Horizontal adductors				
Horizontal abductors				
Internal rotation				
External rotation				
ELBOW AND FOREARM				
Flexors:				
brachioradialis				
biceps				
Extensors				
Supinators				
Pronators				
WRIST				
Flexors:				
flexor carpi ulnaris				
flexor carpi radialis				
Palmaris longus				
Extensors				
Radial deviation				
Ulnar deviation				
FINGERS				
Flexion:				
flexor digitorum profundus				
flexor digitorum sublimis				
lumbricals				
Extensors				
Abductors				
Adductors				

[3] Muscle strength is accurately evaluated when the patient is able to perform isolated movement. The therapist must keep a watchful eye for synergistic substitution patterns, as this can interfere with accurate strength assessment.

Muscle or Muscle group	Tone in supine	Tone in sitting	Tone in standing or walking	Muscle strength grade[3]
THUMB				
Flexor pollicis longus				
Flexor pollicis brevis				
Abductor pollicis				
Opponens pollicis				
Extensors				
LOWER EXTREMITY				
Hip flexors				
Hip extensors				
Hip adductors				
Hip abductors				
Hip internal rotators				
Hip external rotators				
Knee flexors				
Knee extensors				
Ankle plantar-flexors				
Ankle dorsi-flexors				
Ankle inverters:				
midfoot varus				
hindfoot varus				
Ankle everters				
CERVICAL				
TRUNK				

4. ASSESSMENT _____

_____

_____

_____

5. PLAN AND RECOMMENDATIONS (INCLUDING SPECIFIC MUSCLES FOR INJECTION, CASTING, SPLINTING, INHIBITIVE TECHNIQUES, ETC.) _____

_____

_____

_____

_____

Signature _____, OTR

Signature _____, PT

Appendix B
Shriners Hospital for Children
Lexington Unit
Occupational Therapy Rhizotomy Evaluation

Inpatient _____
Outpatient _____

1st evaluation _____ 6 months post-op _____ 1 year post-op _____
Patient Name: _____ Date: _____
Patient Number: _____ Sex: _____
Diagnosis: _____ DOB: _____
Examiner: _____

BIRTH HISTORY:

Age of Gestation _____
Hospitalization _____
Complications _____

DEVELOPMENTAL HISTORY: (at what age did your child do the following)

Roll _____ Sit _____
Stand _____ Walk _____
First word _____ Drink from cup _____
Eat with spoon _____

SOCIAL HISTORY:

Patient lives with _____
School _____
Therapy (OT, PT, ST) _____

COGNITIVE/PSYCHOSOCIAL:

Age appropriate _____ yes _____ no explain _____
Attention/concentration to task _____

COMMUNICATION:

Expressive language
_____ verbal _____ non-verbal
Receptive language
follows simple directions consistently _____ yes _____ no
follows complex directions consistently _____ yes _____ no

ACTIVITIES OF DAILY LIVING: WeeFIM® instrument rating system[1]

No Helper	Helper	
7 = complete independence	5 = supervision	2 = maximal assistance
6 = modified independence	4 = minimal assistance	1 = total assistance
	3 = moderate assistance	

Mobility at home _____

Mobility at school _____

Dressing: (where does child get dressed)

    shirt _____

    shorts _____

    socks _____

    shoes _____

    braces _____

Feeding:

    cup _____

    spoon _____

    fork _____

    knife _____

    set-up _____

    food preparation _____

    clean-up _____

Hygiene/Grooming:

    brushing teeth _____

    combing hair _____

    washing hands _____

    washing face _____

    shaving _____

Bathing: (where does child bathe)

    washing arms _____

    washing legs _____

    washing hair _____

Toileting:

    clothing management _____

    hygiene after toileting _____

    obtain toilet paper/flush toilet _____

Transfers: (sliding board, sit-pivot, stand-pivot)

    bed _____ toilet _____

    bath tub _____ chair _____

Adaptive Equipment:

    w/c _____ walker _____

    tub bench _____ other _____

[1] Copyright © 1993. Uniform Data System for Medical Rehabilitation (UDSMR), a division of UB Foundation Activities, Inc. All rights reserved. Used with permission of UDSMR. All of the marks associated with WeeFIM® belong to Uniform Data System for Medical rehabilitation, a division of UB Foundation Activities, Inc.

Gross Motor Skills:

    roll prone _____   roll supine _____

    ring sit _____   long-leg sit _____

    side sit R_____ L _____   bench sit _____

    crawl _____   push to sit _____

    stand _____   pull to stand _____

    cruise _____   walk _____

    jump _____

Upper Extremity Function:

    hand dominance: right _____ left _____

    contractures right _____ yes _____no measurement _____

               left _____ yes _____no measurement _____

    UE muscle tone (modified Ashworth Scale)

    0 = no increase in tone   1 = slight increase, catch and release

    1+ = slight increase, catch and minimal resistance

    2 = more marked increase through most of range, part easily moved

    3 = considerable increase, passive movement difficult

    4 = parts rigid in flexion or extension

    shoulder flexion R _____ L _____ pronation R _____ L _____

    shoulder extension R _____ L _____ supination R _____ L _____

    shoulder abduction R _____ L _____ wrist flexion R _____ L _____

    shoulder adduction R _____ L _____ wrist extension R _____ L _____

    elbow flexion R _____ L _____ finger flexion R _____ L _____

    elbow extension R _____ L _____ finger extension R _____ L _____

    in-going thumb: right _____ left _____

    reaching overhead: right   _____full _____partial

                      left   _____full _____partial

                    bilateral _____full _____partial

    touch toes: right _____ left _____ bilateral _____

    reach behind back: right _____ left _____

    cross midline: right _____ left _____

    hands to midline: _____

    grip strength: right _____ left _____

    gross grasp (intact right _____ left _____

    release (intact) right _____ left _____

    pinch strength: right   left

       lateral _____

       2-point _____

       3-point _____

       tip _____

    finger isolation: right   left

       index _____

       thumb _____

       little _____

opposition: right   left
thumb to index _____
thumb to middle _____
thumb to ring _____
thumb to little _____
Fine-motor skills: (Peabody)*
   10 beans in bottle: right_____ left_____
   blocks: stacking   right_____ left_____
          train   right_____ left_____
          bridge   right_____ left_____
          steps   right_____ left_____
          pyramid right_____ left_____
Writing Skills: hand used right _____ left _____ both _____
          prehension (Earhardt)_____

horizontal line	vertical line
cross	circle
diagonal line/"X"	name/letters

Assessment/Summary: _____
Strengths: _____
_____
_____
Weaknesses: _____
_____
_____
Plan/Recommendations: _____
_____
_____

* Peabody Developmental Motor Scales and Activity Cards Pro-ed, 8700 Shoal Creek Boulevard, Austin, TX 78757.

Note. The protocols have been developed within the Shriners Hospitals for Children system, for the specific patient population it serves. As a result, Shriners Hospitals for Children cannot make any recommendations or guarantees regarding the propriety of using such protocols for individual patients who are not treated within the Shriners Hospitals for Children system. Reprinted with permission.

Appendix C
Shriners Hospital for Children,
Lexington Unit
Pre Partial Rhizotomy P.T. Assessment

1. GENERAL INFORMATION

Date of Examination ____/____/____ Name of Examiner _____

Name of Patient _____ Sex _____

Date of Birth ____/____/____ Age _____

Diagnosis _____

Parent's Name _____

Address _____ Phone Number _____

2. HISTORY
(Circle source information was gained from: mother, father, medical record, other)

	YES	NO
1. Prematurity BW	____	____
Length of pregnancy in weeks _____		
2. Difficulty in pregnancy	____	____
3. Difficulty with labor	____	____
4. C-section	____	____
5. Difficulty after delivery	____	____
6. Was child jaundiced?	____	____
7. Required transfusion	____	____
8. Was child on respirator or need oxygen	____	____
How long? _____		
9. Length of hospital stay _____		
10. Seizures	____	____

How often _____ When _____

Birth History Comments:

_____

_____

_____

11. In therapy program _____ Started _____

Areas currently being addressed: _____

_____

12. Private Therapist's Name: _____

Address of therapy program: _____

13. School or Developmental Program: name and address: _____

_____

14. Name and address of therapist to do post-op therapy: _____

_____

3. DEVELOPMENTAL HISTORY

(Circle information gained from: parent report, medical record, school record, other)

a. Sit alone on the floor   _____

b. Sit alone on a bench   _____

c. Crawl   _____

d. Get into sitting   _____

e. Pull to stand   _____

f. stand alone   _____

g. walk alone   _____

h. Eat with fingers   _____

i. Feed with a spoon   _____

j. Hold and drink from cup   _____

k. Say daddy and mama appropriately   _____

l. Use 2- and 3-word phrases   _____

4. GENERAL DEVELOPMENT

(Circle information gained from: tester's observation, parent report, medical record)

	YES	NO
a. Speech—age appropriate	____	____
Comments: _____		
b. Intelligence—age appropriate	____	____
Comments: _____		
c. Hand Use—age appropriate	____	____
Comments: _____		
d. Cooperation—age appropriate	____	____
Comments: _____		
e. Hearing—adequate for post-op training	____	____
f. Vision—adequate for post-op training	____	____

5. ORTHOPEDIC PROCEDURES

(Record date and specific type of tenotomy, lengthenings or releases)

a. Gastrocnemius _____   d. Iliopsoas _____

b. Adductors _____   e. Other _____

c. Hamstrings _____

Muscle transfers (describe/date) _____

Hip surgery (describe/date) _____

Derotation osteotomy (describe/date) _____

Foot/ankle surgery (describe/date) _____

Other (describe/date) _____

Muscle Strength/Control Evaluation

Patient Name: _____

Patient #: _____

	ISOLATED STRENGTH		CONTROL	
	RIGHT	LEFT	RIGHT	LEFT
(L1–3) Hip flexors	____	____	____	____
(L5–S2) Hip extensors	____	____	____	____
(L4–S1) Hip abductors	____	____	____	____
(L2–4) Hip adductors	____	____	____	____
(L2–4) Hip internal rotators	____	____	____	____
(L4–S2) Hip external rotators	____	____	____	____
(L2–4) Knee extensors	____	____	____	____
(L5-S2) Knee flexors	____	____	____	____
(L4–S1) Ankle dorsiflexors	____	____	____	____
(L4–S1) Toe extensors	____	____	____	____
(S1–S2) Ankle plantar flexors	____	____	____	____
(L5–S1) Ankle invertors	____	____	____	____
(L5–S1) Ankle evertors	____	____	____	____
(S1–2) Toe flexors	____	____	____	____

Isolated Muscle Scale:

0 = No isolated movement—gravity eliminated

1 = Initiates isolated movement—gravity eliminated

2 = Isolates movement through 1/3 available ROM—gravity eliminated

3 = Isolates movement through 2/3 available ROM—gravity eliminated

4 = Isolates movement through full available ROM—gravity eliminated

5 = Initiates isolated movement—anti-gravity

6 = Isolates movement through 1/3 available ROM—anti-gravity

7 = Isolates movement through 2/3 available ROM—anti-gravity

8 = Isolates movement through full available ROM—anti-gravity

Control Scale:

1 = Unable to isolate motion; no movement

2 = Unable to isolate motion; moves through partial range in pattern

3 = Moves through full range in pattern; takes no resistance

4 = Moves through partial-full range in pattern; takes mild resistance

5 = Moves through partial-full range in pattern; takes moderate resistance

6 = Moves through partial-full range in pattern; takes maximal resistance

7 = Isolates motion; pattern emerges with maximal resistance or stress/effort

Tone Abnormalities
(Tested supine, as resistance to passive stretch)

Patient Name: _____

Patient #: _____

	RIGHT	LEFT
HIP		
Flexors	___	___
Extensors	___	___
Abductors	___	___
Adductors	___	___
External rotators	___	___
Internal rotators	___	___
KNEE		
Flexors	___	___
Extensors	___	___
ANKLE		
Dorsiflexors	___	___
Plantar flexors	___	___
Invertors	___	___
Evertors	___	___
TOE		
Flexors	___	___
Extensors	___	___
ANKLE CLONUS	___	___

Overall tone: _____

_____

_____

*Muscle Tone Scale (Modified Ashworth scale)

0 = No increase in tone

1 = Slight increase, catch and release, or minimal resistance

1+ = Slight increase, catch, and minimal resistance

2 = More marked increase through most of range, parts easily moved

3 = Considerable increase, passive movement difficult

4 = Parts rigid in flexion or extension

POSTURAL REACTIONS:

	RIGHT			LEFT		
	NORMAL	DELAYED	ABSENT	NORMAL	DELAYED	ABSENT
1. Protective reactions in sit:						
Forward	_____	_____	_____	_____	_____	_____
Backward	_____	_____	_____	_____	_____	_____
Sideways	_____	_____	_____	_____	_____	_____
2. Protective reactions in stand:						
Forward	_____	_____	_____	_____	_____	_____
Backward	_____	_____	_____	_____	_____	_____
Sideways	_____	_____	_____	_____	_____	_____
3. Equilibrium in sit (head and trunk)	_____			_____		
4. Equilibrium in stand (head and trunk)	_____			_____		

5. Abnormal Primitive Reflexes _____

_____

_____

MISCELLANEOUS:

1. Clonus at ankles: Right   Left

___ no   ___ no

___ yes   ___ yes

___ # of beats   ___ # of beats

2. Ataxic gait: none _____ slight _____ severe _____

3. Athetoid/ataxic upper extremity movements: none _____ slight _____ severe _____

   Athetoid/ataxic lower extremity movements: none _____ slight _____ severe _____

Comments: _____

_____

_____

_____

Gait (General observations re: pattern, endurance, assistive device, etc.)

_____

_____

_____

_____

Range of Motion

Patient Name: _____

Patient #: _____

	RIGHT	LEFT
HIP		
Flexors	____	____
Extensors	____	____
Abduction (hips extended/flexed)	____	____
Adduction	____	____
Internal/external rotation (hips flexed)	____	____
Internal/external rotation	____	____
Ober test (iliotibial tightness)	____	____
STRAIGHT LEG RAISING	____	____
POPLITEAL ANGLE (from vertical)	____	____
Contralateral knee flexed	____	____
KNEE		
Ely test (rectus femoris tightness)	____	____
Flexion (supine/prone)	____	____
Extension	____	____
Varus/Vagus	____	____
TIBIA		
Torsion (ext or int)	____	____
Rotation (int/ext)	____	____
Thigh/foot angle	____	____
ANKLE		
Dorsiflexion (knee flex/knee ext	____	____
Plantar flexion	____	____
SUBTALAR JOINT		
Inversion/eversion	____	____

HINDFOOT (subtalar neutral)	neutral/varus/valgus	neutral/varus/valgus
FOREFOOT (subtalar neutral)	neutral/varus/valgus	neutral/varus/valgus
FORWARD BENDING ASYMMETRY:	YES/NO	YES/NO
Limb lengths:	R____	L____
ASIS to ASIS	____	

6. EQUIPMENT/APPLIANCES

Type of bracing _____

Type of assistive device(s) _____

Model of wheelchair _____

List seating components on w/c _____
_____

Posture assessment in w/c _____

Wheelchair primarily needed for _____
_____

Describe child's ability to maneuver w/c _____
_____

Method of transferring in/out of w/c _____
_____
_____

Other comments _____

7. SUMMARY

1. Parents goals and expectations from surgery _____
_____
_____
_____

2. Child's goals and expectations from surgery _____
_____
_____

3. Assessment of family support system (as applicable to post-op training) _____
_____
_____

4. Reasons why child is a candidate for selective dorsal rhizotomy (SDR) _____
_____
_____
_____

5. Concerns regarding child's candidacy for SDR surgery _____
_____
_____

Appendix D
Shriners Hospital for Children,
Lexington Unit
Physical Therapy Rhizotomy Video Protocol

AROM: *Supine*—bridging and ankle dorsiflexion with knee extended
　　　Prone—knee flexion
　　　Sidelying—abduction
　　　Sitting—long arc quad

DEVELOPMENTAL ACTIVITIES: Have patient attempt task independently, if necessary, provide assistance. Then have patient hold hands up once position is assumed to test balance and stability in position, if applicable.

　ROLLING: right, Left
　TAILOR SIT
　SIDE SIT: right, Left
　LONG SIT
　QUADRUPED
　CRAWLING
　TALL KNEELING
　KNEE WALKING: forward, right, left, backward
　HALF KNEEL: right, left

COME TO STAND: from 90/90 chair sitting and return to sitting
　　　　　　　from floor to stand and back to floor

90/90 SIT ON CHAIR: with back
　　　　　　　without back

90/90 SIT ON BALL: with upper extremity support
　　　　　　　without upper extremity support
　　　　　　　lateral reaching

TRUNK STRENGTH ON LARGE BALL: flexion unsupine
　　　　　　　　　　　extension unprone

STANDING BALANCE: double stance
　　　　　　　lateral reaching
　　　　　　　heal-to-toe
　　　　　　　single stance: right, left

AMBULATION WITH ORTHOSES:

WALKING:

With assistive device: anterior view
posterior view
lateral view
turning 180°
Without assistive device: anterior view
posterior view
lateral view
stopping
turning 180°
sideways: right, left
backwards—lateral view

RUNNING:

With and without assistive device:
anterior view
posterior view
lateral view

AMBULATION WITHOUT ORTHOSES:

WALKING:

With and without assistive device:
anterior view
posterior view
lateral view

RUNNING:

With and without assistive device:
anterior view
posterior view
lateral view

Appendix E
Shriners Hospital for Children,
Lexington Unit
Shriners Post Rhizotomy Follow-up Physical Therapy Assessment

1. GENERAL INFORMATION

Date of Examination ___ / ___ / ___ Date of Rhizotomy ___ / ___ / _____

Name of Patient _____ Sex _____

Date of Birth ___ / ___ / ___ Age _____

Diagnosis _____

Parent's Name _____

Address _____ Phone Number _____

Name of Examiner _____

2. POST-OP THERAPY

In therapy _____ Started _____

Frequency _____ Has child been consistent in attending therapy? _____

Areas currently being addressed and goals: _____

_____

Therapist's name _____

Address of therapy program _____

_____

School or developmental program. Name and address _____

_____

3. EQUIPMENT/AIDS

Type of bracing _____

Assistive devices _____

Model of wheelchair _____

Seating components on w/c _____

Posture assessment on w/c _____

W/c primarily needed for _____

Method of transferring in and out of w/c _____

4. RANGE OF MOTION

	RIGHT	LEFT
HIP		
Extension (Thomas test)	___	___
Abduction (knees flexed)	___	___
Adduction (knees extended)	___	___
KNEE		
Popliteal angle	___	___
ANKLE		
Dorsiflexion (knee extended)	___	___
Plantar flexion (knee flexed)	___	___

5. STRENGTH

Muscle Strength/Control Evaluation

Patient Name:

Patient #:

	STRENGTH		CONTROL	
	RIGHT	LEFT	RIGHT	LEFT
(L1–3) Hip flexors	——	——	——	——
(L5–S2) Hip extensors	——	——	——	——
(L4–S1) Hip abductors	——	——	——	——
(L2–4) Hip adductors	——	——	——	——
(L2–4) Hip internal rotators	——	——	——	——
(L4–S2) Hip external rotators	——	——	——	——
(L2–4) Knee extensors	——	——	——	——
(L5-S2) Knee flexors	——	——	——	——
(L4–S1) Ankle dorsiflexors	——	——	——	——
(L4–S1) Toe extensors	——	——	——	——
(S1–S2) Ankle plantar flexors	——	——	——	——
(L5–S1) Ankle invertors	——	——	——	——
(L5–S1) Ankle evertors	——	——	——	——
(S1–2) Toe flexors	——	——	——	——

Isolated Muscle Scale:

0 = No isolated movement—gravity eliminated

1 = Initiates isolated movement—gravity eliminated

2 = Isolates movement through 1/3 available ROM—gravity eliminated

3 = Isolates movement through 2/3 available ROM—gravity eliminated

4 = Isolates movement through full available ROM—gravity eliminated

5 = Initiates isolated movement—anti-gravity

6 = Isolates movement through 1/3 available ROM—anti-gravity

7 = Isolates movement through 2/3 available ROM—anti-gravity

8 = Isolates movement through full available ROM—anti-gravity

Control Scale:

1 = Unable to isolate motion; no movement

2 = Unable to isolate motion; moves through partial range in pattern

3 = Moves through full range in pattern; takes no resistance

4 = Moves through partial-full range in pattern; takes mild resistance

5 = Moves through partial-full range in pattern; takes moderate resistance

6 = Moves through partial-full range in pattern; takes maximal resistance

7 = Isolates motion; pattern emerges with maximal resistance or stress/effort

6. TONE

Tone Abnormalities
(Tested supine, as resistance to passive stretch)

Patient Name: _____

Patient #: _____

	RIGHT	LEFT
HIP		
Flexors	____	____
Extensors	____	____
Abductors	____	____
Adductors	____	____
External rotators	____	____
Internal rotators	____	____
KNEE		
Flexors	____	____
Extensors	____	____
ANKLE		
Dorsiflexors	____	____
Plantar flexors	____	____
Invertors	____	____
Evertors	____	____
TOE		
Flexors	____	____
Extensors	____	____
ANKLE CLONUS	____	____

Overall tone: _____

_____

_____

*Muscle Tone Scale (Modified Ashworth scale)

0 = No increase in tone

1 = Slight increase, catch and release, or minimal resistance

1+ = Slight increase, catch, and minimal resistance

2 = More marked increase through most of range, parts easily moved

3 = Considerable increase, passive movement difficult

4 = Parts rigid in flexion or extension

7. ASSESSMENT OF HELP

Activities/exercises performing _____

_____

_____

_____

_____

_____

_____

_____

_____

_____

Frequency _____

Does parent/patient demonstrate appropriately _____

Shriners Post Rhizotomy Follow-up Physical Therapy Assessment

Patient's name:_____

Therapist's name:_____

Address of therapy program _____

_____

Frequency of patient's visits _____

Number of missed visits _____

Compliance of patient with treatment   Good   Fair   Poor

Follow through at home   Good   Fair   Poor

Patient progress/areas currently bing addressed and goals: _____

_____

_____

_____

_____

_____

_____

_____

Therapist recommendations: _____

_____

_____

_____

_____

_____

_____

Questions or concerns from local therapist: _____

_____

_____

_____

_____

Please mail this back to us in the enclosed stamped envelope.

Patient name: _____

Next clinic appointment is: _____

Appendix F
Shriners Hospital for Children,
Lexington Unit
Partial Dorsal Rhizotomy Post-op Treatment in Occupational Therapy

Date Issued: November, 1996   **Policy Number:** OTH514
Department: Occupational Therapy   **Page:** 1 of 2
Signature: _____

	Dates Review/ Revise
	11/96
	2/98

I. POLICY

Those patients who have undergone a partial dorsal Rhizotomy will receive occupational therapy (OT) in accordance with the following treatment protocol:

II. PROCEDURE:

1. Precautions:
    a. Avoid passive trunk rotation for 2 weeks pot-op. Movements should be performed in linear planes. If the child moves actively, rotation is allowed
    b. Support in sitting should be provided with a 90-90-90 alignment, foot rest, and arm support for stability
    c. Make sure the child is placed in a supported position for rest
    d. No aggressive hamstring stretching for 1 week post-op
    e. No hip flexion more than 90 for 2 weeks post-op

2. Treatment Guidelines:

The following treatments are suggested in postoperative care of rhizotomy patients. This is simply a guideline to treatment as each patient must be progressed at his or her individual rate.

Day 3 post-op: Patient begins bedside ROM

    a. Positioning/family education
    b. Total bed rest
    c. Passive range of motion exercises (upper extremity)

Day 8 post-op:

Patient comes to OT department for therapy, which includes tilt table, ROM, transfer training and neurodevelopemental activities, as tolerated

Patient can sit in regular wheelchair, as tolerated

Precautions remain

Day 15 post-op:

Begin upper body dressing/undressing in appropriate plane
Begin pool therapy, to include strengthening, ROM, and standing

OTH514
Page 2 of 2

Discharge Instructions:

If patient receives OT as an outpatient or the school system in their local community, contact with their therapist should be made 2 weeks before discharge. Information regarding expected progress, home program, adaptive equipment and follow-up at Shriners will be relayed by the patient's primary therapist at Shriners Hospital for children.

Provide information to purchase/obtain adaptive equipment. Issue home program to family and arrange other needed services.

Patients are followed-up by OT in the outpatient clinic 6 months and 1 year postoperatively at which times postrhizotomy evaluations will be completed.

Appendix G
Shriners Hospital for Children,
Lexington Unit
Post-op Rhizotomy Care and Follow-up

Date Issued: May, 1996   **Policy Number:** PTH532
Department: Physical Therapy   **Page:** 1 of 2
Signature: _____
Related Departments: _____

	Dates Review/ Revise
1. POLICY	
Patients receiving post-op physical therapy (PT) after partial rhizotomy, shall be treated utilizing the following guidelines:	
	10/96
2. PROCEDURE:	2/97

1. POLICY

Patients receiving post-op physical therapy (PT) after partial rhizotomy, shall be treated utilizing the following guidelines:

2. PROCEDURE:
1. Post-op—5 to 7 days bedrest
   Precautions: Patient to lie prone or in sidelying
2. Day 3—Patient begins bedside active assistive range of motion (AROM) and active range of motion (AROM) to include:
   a. Ankle plantarflexion/dorsiflexion/inversion/eversion
   b. Knee flexion/extension
   c. Hip abduction/adduction/extension/flexion (<90 degrees internal rotation and external rotation.
   Precautions: a. No hip flexion past 90°
   b. No hamstring stretches until 1 week post-op
   c. No passive trunk rotation. If child moves actively, rotation is allowed.
3. Day 8—Patient comes to PT department for therapy which includes strengthening, ROM, stretching, bed mobility, tilt table, transfer and gait training, all as tolerated. May perform hamstring stretches 1 week post-op, to patient's tolerance.
   Precautions: All done to patient's tolerance. No passive hip flexion past 90 degrees or passive trunk rotation for 2 weeks.
4. Day 15—Begin pool therapy to include strengthening (extremities and trunk), ROM< standing and walking activities.
5. Estimated length of stay for ambulatory patients is 4+ weeks; 2 weeks for non-ambulators. This is subject to change depending on patient/family needs, ability to reach goals, and community resources.
6. Discharge goals for ambulatory patients include:
   a. Patient/parents independent in-home program/transfers/gait.
   b. Community ambulators, should be independently ambulatory for 300 feet with appropriate assistive device. Household ambulators should be independently ambulatory for 100 feet with appropriate assistive device.
   c. Patient independent in sit-stand-sit transfers.
   d. Local PT set up as appropriate for patient.

7. Treating therapist should contact local therapist 2 weeks prior to anticipated discharge to discuss follow-up care, locally patients expected progress, home program, adaptive care and follow-up at Shriners.

8. The "Post-op Rhizotomy Follow-up cover Letter" (see attachment 1) is sent to the local therapist, along with the "Local PT Rhizotomy Follow-up Assessment." The therapist is asked to complete this and return prior to patient's return to Clinic.

9. Patients are followed-up at 6 months, 1 year and 2 years postrhizotomy. Stem #6, above, is done one month prior to scheduled RTC, by the Rehab Secretary.

10. Post-op videos are done at 6-month, 1-year, and 2-year intervals, following the rhizotomy video protocol. This should be scheduled along with the RTC appointments.

11. Patients will have a 1 year appointment for gait analysis scheduled by the Motion Analysis Lab personnel at 1 year pot-op.

12. Patients are admitted for six month and one year follow-up. The therapist completes the "Postrhizotomy Follow-Up Assessment" at that time.

Appendix H
Types of Casts

ELBOW AND FOREARM

Drop Out Cast (humeral portion enclosed)

Criteria for Use

- Flexor spasticity or contracture
- Severe contracture (greater than 35–45 degrees)
- Patient in position for gravity to assist (upright)
- Elbow or forearm skin not intact
- Secondary problem requiring mobility at elbow—rheumatoid arthritis (RA), heterotopic ossification (HO)
- Decorticate posturing

Contraindications

- Severely fluctuating tone
- Patient not in position for gravity to assist

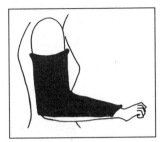

Drop Out Cast (forearm portion enclosed)

Criteria for Use

- Elbow flexor spasticity or contracture
- Severe contracture
- Patient in position for gravity to assist
- Elbow or humeral skin not intact
- Secondary problem requiring mobility
- Decorticate posturing
- May be combined with wrist portion

Contraindications

- Severely fluctuation tone
- Wedging of humeral portion away from arm as elbow extends may be inconvenient or arm may be bound by clothing

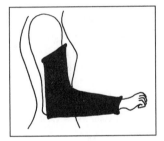

Reverse Drop Out Cast

Criteria for Use

- Elbow extensor spasticity or contracture
- Decerebrate posturing
- Weak biceps may be put at mechanical advantage

Contraindication

- Severely fluctuating tone

Rigid Circular Elbow Cast

Criteria for Use

- Elbow flexor or extensor spasticity or contracture associated with fluctuating tone
- Minimal contracture
- Patient unable to be positioned for optimal drop out cast results

Contraindications

- Skin breakdown at elbow (can "window" cast)
- Severe rigidity
- Secondary problem requiring mobility

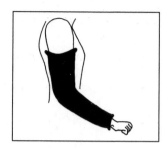

Long Arm Cast (rigid circular elbow, forearm, and wrist cast)

Criteria for Use

- Elbow flexor or extensor contracture associated with supination or pronation contracture
- Elbow and wrist flexor or extensor contracture that must be managed simultaneously

Contraindications

- Skin breakdown at elbow
- Severe rigidity
- Secondary problem requiring mobility

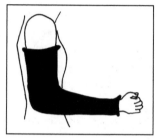

WRIST AND HAND

Rigid Circular Wrist Cast

Criteria for Use

- Wrist flexor or extensor spasticity or contracture
- Full active finger motion in presence of wrist deformity
- Wrist deviation deformity
- Hand function not isolated from wrist function (tenodesis-type hand function with finger extension possible only with wrist flexion)

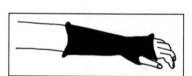

Contraindications

- Subluxation or other orthopedic deformity
- Edema

Rigid Circular Wrist/Metacarpalphalangeal (MP) Cast

Criteria for Use

- Intrinsic musculature of hand spasticity or contracture
- Intrinsics plus position or function

Contraindication

- Severe intrinsic spasticity or contracture in the absence of extrinsic flexor functions may promote proximal interphalangeal (PIP) hyperextension deformity

Rigid Circular Wrist Cast With Thumb Portion

Criteria for Use
- Spasticity in thumb musculature (usually in long flexor)
- Position of thumb effects spasticity in rest of hand

Contraindications
- Subluxation or other orthopedic deformity
- Edema

Rigid Circular Wrist Cast With Finger Shell

Criteria for Use
- Moderate finger flexor spasticity
- Inability to achieve full wrist and finger extension simultaneously, actively, or passively
- Wrist casting alone not effective in promoting further isolation of hand from wrist function

Contraindications
- Severe finger flexor spasticity
- Severe fluctuating tone

Rigid Circular Wrist Cast With Finger Platform

Criteria for Use
- Mild finger flexor spasticity
- Inability to fully extend wrist and fingers simultaneously actively
- Incomplete protection extension pattern in wrist and hand

Contraindication
- Moderate to severe spasticity especially in superficial finger flexors

LOWER EXTREMITY

Long Leg Drop Out Cast (Posterior heel prevents further knee flexion while patient can be ranged into extension)

Criteria for Use

- Stretch heel cord
- Position to promote correct biomechanical alignment for weight bearing
- For splint wear and positioning
- Tone inhibition

Contraindications

- Excessive edema
- Phlebitis
- Be careful of cast slipping on the leg

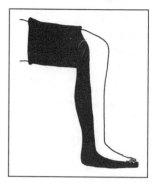

Cylinder Leg Cast

Criteria for Use

- Stretch hamstrings
- Position into knee extension to promote weight bearing in standing
- Prevent skin breakdown behind the knee if contracted and area dampens
- Improve hygiene
- Splint wear
- Tone inhibition

Contraindications

- Excess edema
- Phlebitis
- Excessive hypertension

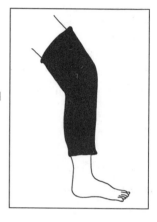

Long Leg Cast (with platform support for toes)

Criteria for Use

- Stretch heel cord
- Position to promote correct biomechanical alignment for weight bearing
- For splint wear/positioning
- Tone inhibition

Contraindications

- Excessive edema
- Phlebitis
- Do not wrap too tight in hip adductor area, because most patients have hypertonicity in adductors

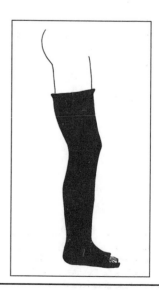

Short Leg Cast

Criteria for Use
- Stretch heel cord
- Position to promote correct biomechanical alignment for weight bearing
- For splint wear and positioning
- Tone inhibition

Contraindications
- Excessive edema
- Phlebitis
- Be careful of pressure on tibial tuberosity

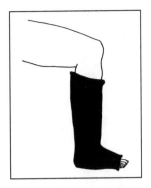

Short Leg Cast With Platform Support for Toes

Criteria for Use
- Stretch heel cord
- Position to promote correct biomechanical alignment for weight bearing
- For splint wear and positioning
- Tone inhibition, in ankle as well as midfoot and hindfoot

Contraindications
- Excessive edema
- Phlebitis
- Be careful of pressure areas around first and fifth metatarsalphalangeal (MTP) heads medial and lateral, respectively.

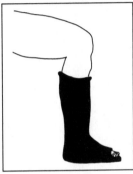

Knee Spreader (can be worn in wheelchair with knees flexed at 90°)

Criteria for Use
- Stretch hip adductors
- To make spreader bar to improve wheelchair sitting

Contraindications
- Excess edema
- Phlebitis
- Excessive hypertension

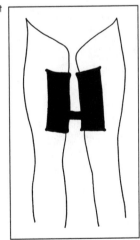

Note. The upper extremity cast drawings are by authors Judy P. Hill, OTR/L and Audrey Yasukawa, MOT, OTR/L, Rehabilitation Institute of Chicago. The lower extremity cast drawings are by Patsy Grooms Cannon, PT, Patricia Neal Rehabilitation Center—Knoxville, TN. All of the drawings were redrawn for purposes of publication in this book by Debra K. Allen.